Supportive and Palliative Care in Cancer

An introduction

Claud Regnard

and

Margaret Kindlen

Radcliffe Medical Press

Radcliffe Medical Press Ltd
18 Marcham Road
Abingdon
Oxon OX14 1AA
United Kingdom

www.radcliffe-oxford.com
The Radcliffe Medical Press electronic catalogue and online ordering facility.
Direct sales to anywhere in the world.

British Library Cataloguing in Publication Data

A catalogue record for this book is available from the British Library.

ISBN 1 85775 937 0

Typeset by Joshua Associates Ltd, Oxford
Printed and bound by Biddles Ltd, Guildford and King's Lynn

Contents

About the authors

Claud Regnard is Consultant in Palliative Medicine, at St Oswald's Hospice, Newcastle City Hospitals NHS Trust and Northgate and Prudhoe NHS Trust, and Honorary Lecturer in Pharmacological Services, University of Newcastle upon Tyne.

Margaret Kindlen is Head of Education, St Oswald's Hospice, Newcastle upon Tyne and Honorary Lecturer, Faculty of Medicine, University of Newcastle upon Tyne. She was previously Senior Lecturer at the Macmillan Education Resource Unit, Department of Medical Education, University of Dundee.

Introduction

In 1995, the Calman–Hine report recommended integration of quality cancer services in England and Wales. It identified gaps in the provision of cancer treatment and variations in the level of competence and experience amongst professionals. The Government responded by establishing a new structure for cancer services throughout the UK. This is based on a network of expertise and the notion of seamless care, which incorporates palliative care into the wider provision of supportive care and treatment of people with cancer. Cancer care is now provided at three levels:

1 Primary care. This is the focus for care.
2 Cancer units. These are large enough to support clinical teams with expertise to manage the more common cancers.
3 Cancer centres. These provide expertise in the management and treatment of common and uncommon cancers within the immediate geographical locality.

The latest development strategy, the NHS Cancer Plan, aims to reduce inequalities of care by:

- boosting prevention and screening services
- in primary care, establishing lead cancer clinicians, funding community nurse training and research
- cutting waiting times and setting up cancer service collaboratives (now part of the NHS Modernisation Agency)
- improving the experience of care through recognising the importance of respect, communication, information, symptom control and psychological support
- improving care through a supportive and palliative care strategy

- establishing guidance on all aspects of palliative and supportive care through NICE (National Institute for Clinical Excellence)
- improving palliative care services through NHS Beacons, the New Opportunities Fund, Palliative Care Networks and improved funding
- establishing cancer and palliative care delivery plans, and setting up a Cancer Nursing Advisory Group to advise on the development of the cancer nursing workforce.

Why an introductory book?

This book is a consequence of the implementation of Calman–Hine and NHS Cancer Plan recommendations. In 1999, The Northern Cancer Network Education subgroup established a framework for cancer and palliative care education based on a competency framework by the Teesside Alliance. This sets a minimum standard of competencies that could be adopted across the region. It became apparent that throughout the region there was adequate education provision to meet higher level proficiency but little to meet the minimum standard of cancer care and palliative care. This introductory book is offered as the first stage of a professional development process. Alongside this book the Northern Cancer Network has commissioned a trainers' pack for a foundation course in cancer and palliative care as the next progressive stage. These provide an adequate basis for the delivery of supportive and palliative cancer care in a non-specialist context.

Who will find the introductory book helpful?

This introductory book has been compiled for staff working in all clinical areas. The aim is to ensure that a common core of information is available to all staff involved in supportive and palliative care for patients with cancer. It is acknowledged and indeed desirable that many members of staff will progress beyond the level of content provided in this introductory book.

How should the introductory book be used

The introductory book can be used either on its own for information and personal learning or as preparation for a foundation course.

- The topics included in this book are thought to be those likely to concern newcomers to cancer and palliative care including non-professional carers.
- For ease of access the topics are arranged in eight sections.
- Information has been confined to just a few pages. Each topic page begins with some information. We have then demonstrated how important the given information is in clinical practice. Finally we offer some key points.
- The last section is a glossary.
- In presenting information in this way we hope that you will have quick access to each topic and have a few essential facts to guide you into good practice in cancer and palliative care.

In the production of this introductory book we have adopted the following definitions:

- It is the right of every person with a life-threatening illness to receive effective supportive care wherever they are.
- It is the responsibility of every healthcare professional to provide effective supportive care, and to call in specialist palliative care colleagues if the need arises, as an integral component of good clinical practice, whatever the illness or its stage.

Supportive care is a vital and integral part of all clinical practice, whatever the illness or its stage, informed by a knowledge and practice of palliative care principles and supported by palliative care specialists. The key principles under-pinning supportive and palliative care should be practised by all healthcare professionals in primary care, hospital and other settings. These are:

- focus on quality of life, which includes good symptom control
- whole person approach, taking into account the person's life experience and current situation
- care which encompasses both the patient and those who matter to that person
- respect for patient autonomy and choice (e.g. over place of care, treatment options, access to specialist palliative care)
- emphasis on open and sensitive communication which extends to patients, informal carers and professional colleagues.

Acknowledgements

The nurse competency framework which prompted this introductory book was adapted by the Northern Cancer Network (NCN) from competencies developed by the Cancer Alliance, Teeside. This book was commissioned by the NCN and financially supported by the North of England Educational Consortium.

We are very grateful to Dr Wendy Makin, Consultant Oncologist and Palliative Medicine Physician, Christie Hospital, Manchester, who edited the cancer aspects of the text. The following sections were written by the NHS Beacon Palliative Care Team, Northgate Hospital (Dorothy Matthews, Lynn Gibson and Claud Regnard), supported by the NHS Executive through the Beacon Awards scheme: Maintaining an environment for eating; How do I help a patient with mouth problems?; What can I do for a patient who does not want to eat or drink?; Identifying distress when communication is poor; Death of a patient's friend or relative; Supporting staff after a patient has died; How can I avoid discrimination?

All other sections were written by Claud Regnard and Margaret Kindlen, supported by a grant through the NCN from the North of England Educational Consortium.

The writers are grateful to the NCN Education Sub Group for their support and comments:

Ingrid Ablett-Spence   Elaine Kilganon
Shirley Edgar   Margaret Kindlen
Sandra Gaines   Shaun Kinghorn
Richard Gamlin   Shirley Richardson
Kath Henderson   Jill Starkey

Claire Huddart   Helen Tucker
Joan James   Jimmy Youill

Finally, the writers would particularly like to thank Shirley Edgar, Shirley Richardson and Ingrid Ablett-Spence whose support ensured that the introductory book was completed.

Section 1
Cancer

- What is cancer?
- What causes cancer?
- Types of cancer
- Detecting cancer
- Cancer diagnosis and monitoring

What is cancer?

What should I know?

Cancer is a group of diseases. Cancers can arise from any of the normal tissues in the body, therefore there can be many different types of cancer. The two hallmarks of cancers are their ability for uncontrolled growth and their potential to invade other tissues.

How common is cancer?

Forty percent (2 in 5) of the population will be affected by cancer. Some cancers are much more common than other cancers.

How serious is a diagnosis of cancer?

Twenty-five percent (1 in 4) of the population will die from cancer. Many cancers can be cured, especially if diagnosed at an early stage. Other cancers present late or are resistant to treatment.

Uncontrolled growth

The ability of cells to grow and reproduce is normally tightly controlled to ensure the body maintains its correct shape and function. Occasionally a cell will grow and duplicate itself with little control. If it stays as a local lump this is called a benign tumour. It only becomes a cancer if it has the potential to spread.

The potential for spread

Unlike other cells, cancer cells can spread from their original site (the 'primary tumour') by invading local tissues or spreading to distant sites ('secondary tumours' or 'metastases').

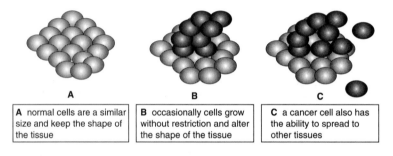

A	**B**	**C**
A normal cells are a similar size and keep the shape of the tissue	**B** occasionally cells grow without restriction and alter the shape of the tissue	**C** a cancer cell also has the ability to spread to other tissues

Treatment and progress of cancer

Cancer treatment can include surgery, radiotherapy or chemotherapy, or a combination of these to eradicate cancer cells.

Following treatment some tumour cells may survive and subsequently cause problems for patients through local recurrence or metastatic spread.

Local recurrence

The microscopic cells that are not killed by original treatment continue to grow at the original primary site and eventually give rise to symptoms. Most recurrences appear within 1–2 years after initial treatment, although sometimes it takes many years before they appear.

Metastatic spread

Cancer cells spread in two ways.

- **Local spread**: a cancer can invade nearby tissues causing damage or distortion of those tissues.
- **Distant spread**: cells can break off from the primary tumour to form satellite sites. This process is called 'metastatic spread'. The cancer cells can spread through lymph or blood vessels. Common sites of metastases include lymph nodes, bone, lungs and liver.

The pattern of spread varies between different cancers.

How can I use this information?

Knowing the typical pattern of spread of a cancer indicates where to look for signs of local or distant spread (see Table below).

Cancer type	Local recurrence	Metastatic spread
Lung cancer	Lymph nodes in chest	Common in late stages, especially to bone, liver and brain
Breast cancer	Breast, skin of chest wall, or lymph nodes in armpit	Bone, lung, liver and brain (but may occur after a delay of several years)
Large bowel (colon) cancer	Abdominal cavity	Liver and lung

Key points

- Cancer can arise from any normal tissue in the body.
- The two hallmarks of cancer are uncontrolled growth, and the ability of the original site (the primary tumour) to spread to other tissues.
- Spread of cancer can be by the invasion of nearby tissues, and by spreading to distant tissues through the blood or lymphatic system (metastatic spread) to form secondary tumours or metastases.
- Different cancers have different patterns of spread.

What causes cancer?

What should I know?

There is no single cause of cancer but there are many factors that combine to increase the risk. There are two types of factor – those that are within the individual and others that are external. For many people, cancer will only develop if several factors are present.

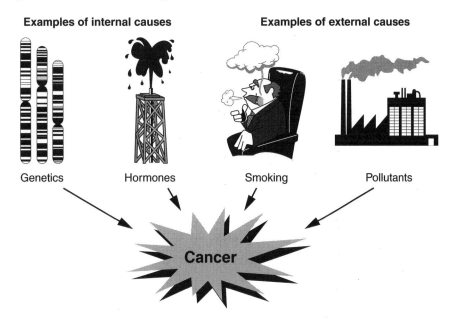

Examples of internal causes **Examples of external causes**

Genetics   Hormones   Smoking   Pollutants

Cancer

Internal factors

Genetics: we inherit our characteristics through our genes passed on from our parents. For most people there is no obvious hereditary cause of cancer. However, we now know that many people with cancer have a basic change in the cell genes which control normal growth. It is this fault which leads to the development of cancer. Cancer is inherited in a few people, but this type of inheritance is rare, e.g. less than 5% of all breast cancer cases originate from detectable genetic abnormalities.

Hormones: although hormones can affect the growth of cancer, very few cancers are caused by natural hormones (cancer of the uterus is one such type). Some cancers are sensitive to changes in hormones and this sensitivity is used in the treatment of breast and prostate cancers.

External factors

Exposure to environmental factors over a period of time can cause cancer. Tobacco tars are the biggest cause of cancer, but many chemicals, viruses and physical agents (e.g. ultraviolet light in sunlight) can have a similar effect. This has implications for work-related cancers resulting from exposure to asbestos, soot, some metals, radiation or sunlight.

Each of these agents has a particular association with a particular type of cancer, e.g. tobacco with lung cancer, oesophageal and bladder cancer; and ultraviolet light/sunlight with skin cancer.

However, it is important to realise that there are often several causes. Several of these factors are needed together to affect the way some cells grow and reproduce.

How can I use this information?

Knowing what factors might increase the risk of cancer will help you recognise how certain lifestyles and work histories are important.

Industry and organisations where there are potential hazards relating to materials being used are subject to health and safety standards and are required to monitor the health of the workforce.

Family doctors when aware of family history of a specific cancer will be on the alert and channel people into screening programmes.

Key points

- There is no single cause of cancer.
- A combination of genetic faults and exposure to external agents causes most cancers.

Types of cancer

What should I know?

Tissues that are the source of cancer

Cancer can develop from any cell in the body, therefore the range of cancers is large – there are over 200 types of cancer. However, there are only four types of cells that can be the source of cancer.

- **Surface or lining (epithelial) tissues:**
  - skin
  - the lining of tubes and cavities (such as the bowel)
  - the tissues that make up glands (such as the breast). These types of cancer are called a carcinoma, and those developing from glands are known as an adenocarcinoma.
- **Internal tissues:** these include the tissues that make bone, muscle, fat and other soft tissues.
- **Blood and lymphatic tissues:** these consist of the blood, bone marrow, lymph nodes and spleen. The lymphatic tissues and part of our blood form our immune system that fights infection.
- **Neurological tissues:** these include the brain, eyes, spinal cord and nerves.

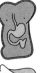

Surface or lining tissues, e.g. skin, bowel

Internal tissues, e.g. bone, fat

Blood and lymphatic tissues

Neurological tissues

The similarity of cancer cells to normal cells

Normal cells are well organised in that they do the correct job, grow in the right place to the right shape and size, and respond to signals to stop reproducing. Cancer cells vary in the extent to which they resemble a normal cell.

- **Differentiated cancer cells**: these are cells that look and function like normal cells. Tumours made up from these cells tend to grow more slowly, giving more time for treatment to take effect.
- **Undifferentiated cancer cells**: these cells have very little in common with the normal cells they came from, and tend to grow in a disorganised, haphazard fashion. Tumours made up from these cells tend to grow more quickly and be less predictable in the way that they grow and spread, making treatment more difficult.
- **Stem cells**: these are cells that have the ability to change into several different types of cells. They are found in the early embryo stages of development and in the bone marrow. Cancers developing from these stem cells may stay undifferentiated or become more differentiated.

Primary and secondary cancers (metastases)

The original cancer is known as the *primary cancer*. Cancers can spread to other tissues as 'metastases'; these are *secondary cancers*. These are not different cancers; the cells are usually the same as the primary cancer. Even large secondary cancers start as single cancer cells breaking off from the primary cancer and spreading through tissues, blood vessels or lymph vessels to other tissues.

How can I use this information?

Skin cancers

These comprise:

- those that remain localised and grow very slowly, e.g. solar keratosis
- those that invade skin and may ulcerate, e.g. basal cell carcinoma
- those that invade skin and surrounding tissues and may form metastases in local lymph nodes, e.g. squamous cell carcinoma
- those that start in the skin but can spread rapidly to many different tissues, e.g. melanoma.

Lining of tubes, cavities and glands

Examples are cancers of the bowel, cervix and lung. Because of their position they may show early signs of their presence and may be cured by early removal. If they are not found, cancers in the abdomen tend to spread to the liver, while others spread to nearby tissues and lymph nodes. Breast cancer is the most common cancer in women and can be cured if found early. At a later stage it spreads to nearby tissues, local lymph nodes and to bone. Many linings contain glands, so that cancers of the bowel, cervix and breast are known as adenocarcinomas. Lung cancer can develop from a lining without glands (e.g. a bronchial carcinoma) or one with glands (e.g. lung adenocarcinoma).

Cancers of internal tissues

Cancers of bone, muscle, fat or other soft tissues tend to occur in children or young people and are uncommon or rare. The usual type is called a sarcoma, e.g. osteosarcoma, a sarcoma of the bone. They tend to grow and spread rapidly.

Blood and lymphatic tissues

The cancers of the lymphatic tissues, e.g. Hodgkin's lymphoma. These tend to affect many lymph nodes in the body as well as the spleen, liver and bone marrow.

The cancers of the blood:
• myeloma, where one type of cell in the blood, the plasma cells, produce too much of a special protein usually used to fight infection
• the leukaemias, a cancer of the white cells that fight infection; they vary from rapidly developing forms in children, to very slowly growing forms in old age.

Neurological cancers

In children, these are rare but can be a rapidly growing cancer of the brain, eye or other parts of the nervous system. In adults they tend to occur in the brain and their growth can be very slow in some, or very fast in other types. Such cancers in the central nervous system do not usually spread outside into other tissues.

Key points

- Cancer types are defined by the cell of origin, and how differentiated the cells are compared with normal cells.
- Some cancers do not spread, some spread at an early stage, while some spread at a late stage.
- Different cancers grow at different rates.

Detecting cancer

What should I know?

Early diagnosis and treatment for cancer increases the likelihood of cure. Unfortunately many of the symptoms associated with the early stages of cancer are vague, often felt to be unimportant and are consequently ignored. Another difficulty is that many of the early warning signs of cancer may have other causes.

In 1983 The American Cancer Society provided an reminder – **CAUTION** – as a way of giving some guidance to the public about important signs that should prompt them to seek medical advice. **CAUTION** stands for:

C

A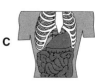

U

T

I

O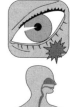

N

Change in bladder or bowel habit
A sore which does not heal
Unusual bleeding or discharge
Thickening or lump in breast or elsewhere
Indigestion or difficulty in swallowing
Obvious change of a wart or mole
Nagging cough or persistent hoarseness.

Many breast and testicular lumps are discovered accidentally and through self-examination. In the UK the Government has promoted early detection of cancer and has supported campaigns through NHS-funded and National Cancer Charities to encourage public awareness in self-examination techniques.

Looking for early signs combined with self-examination techniques is a way of screening ourselves.

Cancer screening

Cancer screening programmes aim to detect early cancer or the changes that occur in tissues before cancer develops. These are aimed at a healthy population who are in the age group most commonly affected by a particular cancer. The features of an effective screening programme are that:

- early treatment must be offered that will reduce the mortality rate of the disease
- the tests offered must be reliable and accurately diagnose early disease
- the screening programme must be able to help high-risk groups
- whenever possible offer treatments that are simple and well tolerated
- the screening programme must have an effective and fail–safe communication and recall system.

For many cancers, tests are not yet sensitive enough, so that cancers are picked up too late to make any difference to survival. However, three types of cancer are amenable to mass screening.

Cervical cancer

The cervical smear test has proved to be an accurate and reliable test to detect cervical cancer at an early stage of cervical cancer and can even detect changes that occur before cancer starts. Many women have been diagnosed before any signs or symptoms have presented. However, women still die from this disease either because some cervical cancers are very aggressive at the time of diagnosis, or because some women do not get screening.

Breast cancer

The fact that this cancer is curable if detected and treated early has driven the increase in cancer screening services available to women. Screening saves over 600 lives each year in the UK alone. Breast self-examination is simple and can be carried out privately. It should be done as soon as the menstrual period has finished since breasts are less likely to feel lumpy at this time.

Testicular cancer

This occurs in younger men and is potentially curable. A programme has recently started to encourage men to examine their testicles after a warm bath or shower to check for unusual lumps or pain.

How can I use this information?

Following the Forrest Report[1] all women in the UK between 50 and 64 years of age are offered mammography every three years. Mammography is a soft tissue X-ray of the breast, nipple and overlying skin. It enables the radiologist to see different views of the breast from different angles.

Some women find the screening embarrassing and uncomfortable. You might find yourself in a situation with a woman who is considering not attending for a first or subsequent examination. Whilst this is ultimately the person's own choice you can explain how important this investigation is. Knowing it to be a potentially uncomfortable and embarrassing experience, you can be sympathetic, supportive and positive.

If a lump is detected at the time of screening, a procedure called 'fine needle aspiration' will be carried out in which a tiny sample of cells and fluid are drawn from the lump and sent off for examination under a microscope.

Key points

- Early signs of cancer are difficult to detect and to a large extent depend on patient self-reporting.
- Self-examination techniques can help speed up the process of early diagnosis.
- Screening programmes are available to assist the early detection of breast and cervical cancer.

---

1   Forrest P, Sir and Working Group on Breast Cancer Screening (1987) *Breast Cancer Screening: Report to Health Ministers of England, Wales, Scotland and Northern Ireland.* The Stationery Office, London.

Cancer diagnosis and monitoring

What should I know?

A wide range of tests can now be used to diagnose cancer, assess its extent, and monitor its progress.

How can I use this information?

Any test provokes anxiety in a patient and they will need the opportunity to safely express their concerns. They will need to know what happens during each test. The unknown can be frightening and explaining the procedure makes the test easier. Below is a description of the most common investigations.

Biopsy

This involves taking a piece of the suspicious tissue for analysis. A needle biopsy may be done through a short needle or a longer needle (perhaps using a special scan for guidance e.g. CT or ultrasound). Biopsies can be taken at endoscopy (*see* p. 19) or occasionally tissue is taken during an operation.

Procedure (needle biopsy): the patient lies down. The skin over the area to be biopsied is cleaned and numbed with local anaesthetic. With a short needle tissue is simply sucked through into a syringe. With longer needles time is taken to ensure the correct spot is found, and then with a 'click' the needle cuts out a small piece of tissue.

X-rays

These are used routinely in the screening for breast cancer, but will also show the common lung cancers. It can be useful in checking for the presence of any spread to bone, but small deposits will not show. Other tissues are not easily seen.

Procedure: the patient stands or lies down. Each picture only takes seconds.

CT and MRI scans

CT uses X-rays taken from many angles. These are analysed by computer to produce a detailed image of most tissues. MRI uses the effect of strong magnetic fields on tissues to give much more detailed pictures than CT. Both are used to see the extent of tumour spread before surgery or radiotherapy, or to monitor the effect of treatment.

Procedure: the patient lies down and is gently slid into a doughnut-shaped machine. The machine makes a clanking sound as it operates, taking up to 20 minutes to build up a picture. It may be necessary to inject a dye into a vein to improve the pictures.

Ultrasound

This uses high frequency sound waves to see into the body. The sound waves are directed at the area to be examined. The reflected sound waves are used to build up a picture of the internal structures. Detail is poor but its simplicity is useful in early tests, especially of the abdomen. It is also used in detecting blood clots in the legs.

Procedure: the patient lies down. A little jelly is placed on the skin over the area to be examined. A probe is then slid over the skin to build up a picture of the area beneath.

Radioisotopes

These are short-acting radioactive chemicals attached to molecules which will attach to specific tissues. The radiation they give off can then be seen by detectors.

It is most commonly used to detect new bone formation caused by spread of the cancer to bones. It can detect small deposits anywhere in the skeleton.

Procedure: the patient is given the radioisotope by intravenous injection a few hours before the procedure. At the time of the scan the patient lies down and a flat, circular, scanning instrument slowly moves up and down the body. The scan is complete in 15–20 minutes.

Cancer markers

Some tumours produce chemicals that are specific to one type of cancer. These chemicals can be used to screen for some cancers, to monitor the effects of treatment and to detect any return of the cancer. Cancers of the prostate, ovary and bowel are monitored in this way.

Procedure: a simple blood test.

Endoscopy

This usually uses narrow, flexible telescopes which can be inserted into the mouth or rectum to inspect the throat, gullet, stomach, bowel, bladder, airway and lungs. Rigid telescopes can be inserted through the skin of the abdomen to look inside the abdominal cavity.

Procedure: the patient lies down. They are given sedation when it is necessary to look at the airway, lungs or abdomen. For other areas the telescope is gently inserted into the mouth and swallowed, or gently inserted into the rectum. Biopsies can be taken through the endoscope. The procedure takes 15–20 minutes.

Key points

- A wide range of tests can now be used to diagnose cancer, assess its extent, and monitor its progress.
- Explaining what happens during a test makes it less frightening.
- Many tests take no more than 20 minutes.

Section 2
Cancer treatments

- How is a cancer treatment chosen?
- Surgery
- Radiotherapy: overview
- Radiotherapy: side effects
- Chemotherapy: overview
- Chemotherapy: side effects
- Hormone therapy

How is cancer treatment chosen?

What should I know?

Choosing the right treatment for cancer is crucial to ensure as many patients as possible are cured, or at least have a prolonged survival.

Choosing treatment depends on a number of factors:

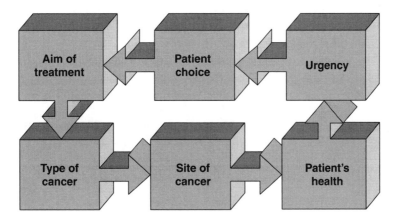

Aim of treatment: the stage of the disease will indicate whether cure is possible or the aim is to control symptoms. For example, if a cancer is localised to where it started it will be easier to remove by surgery, whereas if it has spread (as metastases) then treatments that travel throughout the bloodstream may be chosen such as chemotherapy.

Type of cancer: this may decide which treatment is best since some cancers respond better to one type of treatment.

Site: this will decide whether treatments such as surgery or radiotherapy can be used.

General health of the patient: clearly a very ill patient will not tolerate some treatments as well as a relatively fit patient.

Urgency: conditions such as compression of the spinal cord need a quick-acting treatment such as radiotherapy or surgery.

Patient choice: sometimes there is more than one way of treating a cancer. For example, in breast cancer removal of the lump may give the same result as removing all the breast (mastectomy), but with the right information patients may choose one over the other.

How can I use this information?

Breast cancer: early breast cancer can be treated with removal of the breast lump and possibly removal of some lymph nodes. This avoids mastectomy, but radiotherapy to the breast must be given. If any lymph nodes have cancer in them then the neck and armpit (axilla) are treated with radiotherapy to prevent the cancer returning locally. Chemotherapy is being offered to patients to reduce the risk of the cancer returning. Since breast cancers can be dependent on the female hormone oestrogen, drugs which reduce the effect of oestrogen are also used.

Breast cancer
Surgery, radiotherapy,
chemotherapy,
hormones

Cancer of the lung: removal of all or part of the lung with surgery is the first choice if the tumour is sufficiently localised. This may be followed by radiotherapy to the site of the cancer. If the tumour cannot be removed then radiotherapy alone is used. Chemotherapy is best for some lung cancers.

Prostate cancer: early prostate cancer is treated with surgery or radiotherapy to the pelvis. Often there is spread to the bones at the time the cancer is detected, but since prostate cancers can be dependent on the male hormone androgen, drugs which reduce its effect are used. Radiotherapy is very useful in treating bone pain but, in contrast, chemotherapy is not very effective.

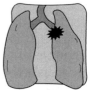

Cancer of lung
Surgery, radiotherapy,
chemotherapy

Cancer of the cervix: screening programmes are able to find and detect very small cancers, or cells at risk of turning into cancer. These are treated by local removal of the abnormal cells. Early cancers require surgery or radiotherapy. In these cases radiotherapy is given using sources of radiation external to the body, or inserted close to the cervix. Radiotherapy can successfully treat even advanced cancers that are localised to the pelvis. Chemotherapy can be an option for someone in whom the cancer has spread.

Bowel cancer: when it is found early enough, surgical removal is usually curative. Chemotherapy is reserved for those who are found at diagnosis to have cancer that has spread to other organs and areas. In cancers of the rectum, radiotherapy and surgery are used together, or radiotherapy is used alone if the cancer is too advanced to be removed.

Choosing treatments for the complications of cancer

Bone metastases: when cancer spreads to bone this can cause pain and fractures. Radiotherapy gives good pain relief in 80% of patients treated. Drugs can also be used that encourage bone healing, while surgery can be used if a fracture is a risk or has already happened.

Compression of the spinal cord: if this is not treated it will result in paralysis below the point of damage. Patients are given steroids to reduce the swelling around the cord and urgent radiotherapy is arranged. Occasionally surgery is needed if steroids and radiotherapy have failed.

Obstructed bowel: surgery is the treatment of choice, but if patients are too ill for surgery, symptom control can be effective enough to keep patients at home if they wish.

Brain metastases: spread of cancer to the brain may cause local problems with brain function such as local weakness, or they can increase pressure in the skull causing headaches, nausea and vomiting. Steroids can be used to reduce any swelling around the brain followed by radiotherapy.

Key points

- Treatment for cancer is individualised to patients.
- Different cancers requires different approaches, often with combinations of treatment.
- Complications of cancer also require specific combinations of treatment.

Surgery

What should I know?

In the early days of cancer treatment, surgery was the only option. Today surgery is still a key part of cancer management.

Types of cancer surgery

Diagnosis and assessment: investigations can often confirm the presence and extent of cancer, but sometimes surgery is the only way to obtain tissue to establish the type and extent of the cancer. (See *Cancer diagnosis and monitoring*, pp. 17–19.)

Curative surgery: if the cancer is localised to one organ or area, it will be possible to remove the cancer before it has spread. In many cases tissue around the cancer is removed. This may include local lymph glands in case the cancer has spread to them. Occasionally removal of tissue and glands has to be extensive to reduce the risk of the tumour returning, e.g. removing a breast (mastectomy).

Treatment surgery: if surgery is not possible, radiotherapy or chemotherapy are used to reduce the size of the tumour which can then be removed with surgery. Alternatively, limited surgery can be done, with radiotherapy or chemotherapy being given later. This type of surgery means less damage is done to appearance and function.

Emergency surgery: occasionally surgery is needed to correct emergencies such as a compressed spinal cord that has not responded to radiotherapy, a blocked bowel, or a fractured bone.

Palliative surgery: surgery is useful in easing symptoms or preventing future problems, even though it is not possible to cure the cancer. Examples are removing an ulcerated tumour or placing a metal pin in a bone to relieve pain or prevent a fracture.

Reconstructive surgery: this is used to restore function or appearance to an area that has been removed or altered. Examples are plastic surgery after head and neck cancer or breast reconstruction after mastectomy. This surgery is usually performed after cancer treatment has finished, but it can be done at the time of the original surgery.

The side effects of surgery

Patients have to make both physical and psychological adjustments to surgery. For example, some surgery is simple and requires only a brief general anaesthetic, such as bypassing a bowel obstruction by making a simple colostomy. Physical recovery from such surgery will be rapid, but it may take the patient longer to adjust to having a colostomy. Other surgery is much more complex and requires a long recovery period, but the benefits may mean the patient adjusts sooner.

Surgical action	Examples of side effects of surgery
General anaesthetic and tissue damage	Fatigue, weight loss, stress, risk of infection
Removal of visible structure, e.g. breast, testes	Loss or difficulty with body image
Removal of functioning tissue, e.g. thyroid, bowel, muscle	Need for replacement drugs, altered diet, altered function
Nerve damage	Impotence, pain, muscle paralysis
Formation of external opening, e.g. colostomy	Loss or difficulty with body image, difficulty coping with new procedures

How can I use this information?

Psychological: patients who have just had emergency surgery may have no idea that a cancer has been discovered. Others may have surgery before they have had time to adjust to their diagnosis. Both will need permission to express their feelings safely. Most patients guess something is seriously wrong within days. The duty of professionals is to find out if they want to discuss their situation further, not to decide what they should be told. (See *What about breaking bad or difficult news?*, pp. 110–13.)

Physical: patients will need physical help with washing, eating, drinking and toiletting after complex surgery. Observing for signs of infection and other problems is important. Distraction of their choice (TV, radio, music, reading, visitors) becomes important as they improve. A quiet environment is more comfortable for some patients, but others prefer company in open bays or wards.

Recovery: as a patient recovers they will need to relearn mobility and independence, and some will need to adapt to a change in their function or body image. This period is as crucial as the time just after surgery since it will influence how well the patient adjusts in the future.

At every stage, being positive is important. Most of the effects of surgery are temporary or respond to treatment, but fatigue and adjusting to change will take longer. You need to be aware of the effects of surgery and report or encourage the patient to report anything that is not normal for them.

Key points

- Surgery still has a key role in cancer treatment.
- Some surgery is simple with rapid recovery.
- Patients receiving more complex surgery will need time and support to re-adapt to changed function or body image.

Radiotherapy: overview

What should I know?

Radiotherapy is an effective treatment for many types of cancer. It uses high energy X-rays to kill off cancer cells. However, these also damage normal cells so the aim in radiotherapy is to get maximum radiation to cancer cells without too much damage to normal ones. To achieve this the dose of radiotherapy must be carefully calculated and the exact area to be irradiated must be carefully planned. Radiotherapy also includes the controlled use of radioactive materials which release radiation similar to X-rays.

The dose of radiotherapy and the number of treatments given are dependent on the purpose for which the radiotherapy is being used.

- **Curative**, which is used as the main treatment for cancer.
- **Treatment** used in conjunction with surgery to remove cancer cells that have spread and could cause the cancer to restart. This is also called 'adjuvant' treatment.
- **Palliative treatment** used to treat distressing symptoms of advanced cancer and to enhance quality of life.
- **Emergency treatment** used in situations such as compression of the spinal cord, blockage of a main vein by tumour, severe pain or bone damage that is risking or causing a fracture.

Generally speaking radiotherapy dosage is higher and the treatment takes longer when cure is the aim. Lower doses in one or two sessions are used when symptom control is the main aim.

How does radiotherapy work?

Normal cells reproduce in response to the death of other cells, thus maintaining a constant number of cells in the body. Cells divide at different rates. Cells such as cancer cells that have rapid rates of cell division are more sensitive to radiation. Some normal cells in the body also divide rapidly and can be affected by radiotherapy. These include bone marrow; lymphatic tissue; epithelial lining of the gastrointestinal and genitourinary tracts; ovaries and testes; and skin and hair follicles.

How is radiotherapy given?

Radiotherapy is usually given on an outpatient basis.

Dose: the measurement unit for radiotherapy is the 'Gray'. The total dose will depend on how sensitive the cancer cell is to radiotherapy and whether the aim of the treatment is curative, adjuvant or palliative. The sensitivity of surrounding tissue also needs to be taken into account. The oncologist prescribes a dose which will effectively kill the cancer without too much damage to healthy tissue.

Divided doses: this is called 'fractionation' and is an important part of curative and treatment radiotherapy. The total dose is divided into 'fractions' given daily. Because cancer cells recover more slowly than normal cells, fewer cancer cells survive with each fraction, while damage to surrounding tissues is kept to a minimum.

Fields: this is the area that receives the radiotherapy. Each fraction of radio-therapy is given from a different angle over a period of days or weeks. By changing the angle and direction, different areas of healthy tissue are exposed to radiotherapy whilst the cancer cells are subjected to repeated blows. Once the treatment fields have been determined, the total area to be treated is marked on the skin with a purple dye.

Radiotherapy is delivered in different ways, for example:

External beam therapy from a machine called a linear accelerator sends a carefully directed beam of X-rays to the tumour area. The patient lies on a couch under the machine.

Sealed unit radioactive sources: these may be needles which are inserted into, or near, a tumour. The advantage is that the radiotherapy is delivered very close to the tumour with little effect on surrounding tissues.

Unsealed sources are radioisotopes in liquid or solid form given by injection, drink or placed inside an organ of the body. For example radioactive strontium may be given as a injection to patients with prostate cancer. The strontium is taken up by bone metastases where it kills off the cancer cells.

How can I use this information?

The reactions or side effects to radiotherapy are relative to the site being treated. A patient having radiotherapy to the rectum may experience some diarrhoea. Similarly, radiotherapy to the scalp will result in temporary loss of hair. The most common side effects of radiotherapy are tiredness and fatigue. These are discussed in the next section.

Your role in supporting a person receiving radiotherapy is to listen and respond to any concerns that arise directly or indirectly from the treatment or indeed to the knowledge that they have cancer.

Key points
- Radiotherapy is one of the recognised treatments for many types of cancer.
- Radiotherapy may be given as a curative or palliative treatment.
- The most common side effects of radiotherapy are tiredness and fatigue.

Radiotherapy: side effects

What should I know?

Most treatment in advanced cancer is palliative – doses are lower and therefore side effects are mild or absent. Higher doses are needed in curative or adjuvant treatment and short-term and long-term side effects can be more troublesome.

Skin

Skin exposed to radiotherapy can become pink, and later become red, swollen and sore (this is called inflammation). With modern techniques, however, skin reactions are mild or absent. The exception to this is when the skin itself is being treated. Although this can cause the surrounding skin to become raw, moist and sore, healing occurs quickly once the treatment has finished.

How can you help? The skin within the treatment area can be safely cleaned by gentle washing with tepid water. Soap should not be used and the skin should always be patted dry with a soft towel. Baby dusting powder can be used and the treatment area should not be shaved during treatment. The dye marks that provide the guide for treatment should remain until treatment is complete. A gentle steroid cream is sometimes used to reduce inflammation.

Tiredness and fatigue

Patients receiving radiotherapy commonly feel tired. It usually begins in the first week of treatment, reaches a peak after 2 weeks and gradually reduces a few weeks after treatment is completed. An intensive course of radiotherapy should be thought of as the equivalent of a major operation and patients need to rest and take things easy afterwards. Unlike surgery, it may take several weeks for the benefits of radiotherapy to become apparent.

Other side effects

Remembering that radiotherapy affects both the cancer and the surrounding tissues, there will be particular symptoms associated with different areas treated. These are listed in the table below.

It is worth remembering that

- side effects depend on the radiation dose and area treated
- palliative radiotherapy often has very few or no side effects
- many side effects are effectively treated or settle when treatment ends.

Area treated	Possible side effects of radiotherapy
Brain	Hair loss (alopecia) is the main side effect, but the hair starts to re-grow within weeks of stopping treatment
Head and neck	Dryness of the mouth and throat; alterations in taste and inflammation of the lining of the mouth, throat and gullet
Abdomen and lower back	Nausea and vomiting (but only if upper abdomen is treated), diarrhoea and bladder inflammation occur 10–14 days after treatment (if pelvis is treated) and can last several weeks
Lymph nodes	Damage to lymph channels causes an accumulation of lymph in tissues causing a swollen limb (lymphoedema)

How can I use this information?

You might be involved in preparing a patient to receive radiotherapy. You might observe some of the effects mentioned above and you may be involved in treating side effects or rehabilitating a patient following treatment.

Frequently patients begin treatment before they have had time to take on board what is happening to them. In these circumstances patients do not always hear what is being said. So you might be faced with a frightened patient who does not understand what is happening or think that they have not been told what is happening to them.

They may have misconceptions about radiotherapy. In most cancer centres there are specialist nurses available in the radiotherapy department to help patients who are having major difficulties coming to terms with their diagnosis and treatment plan. Your involvement might be to listen and, when appropriate, encourage the patient to ask questions or to reveal their concerns to the doctor or other professional.

Being positive is important. Most of the effects of treatment are temporary and respond to treatment. You therefore need to be aware of and on the alert for the effects of treatment and report or encourage the patient to report anything that is not normal for them.

Key points

- Most effects of radiotherapy are restricted to the area being treated.
- Frequently patients begin treatment before they have had time to come to terms with their diagnosis.
- Most of the effects of treatment are temporary and respond to treatment.

Chemotherapy: overview

What should I know?

Chemotherapy simply means drug treatment. Cancer chemotherapy usually means using drugs that can kill cancer cells. There are many different cancer chemotherapy drugs available so treatments can be very different. They all have the advantage of reaching nearly all parts of the body.

Many cancers respond to chemotherapy. However, only a small proportion of cancers can be cured with chemotherapy alone and these include many of the cancers of the blood (leukaemias), lymph nodes (e.g. lymphoma), and some childhood cancers. Treatment of most other cancers uses chemotherapy in combination with surgery or radiotherapy, especially if there is a high risk of secondary spread. Chemotherapy also has a role in treating cancers that have already spread beyond the primary tumour.

Cancer chemotherapy aims to kill cancer cells, but it also kills normal cells, so the aim is to have the maximum effect on the cancer while keeping damage to normal cells to a minimum. To achieve this the drugs, doses and number of treatments are selected for each individual who is regularly monitored throughout the treatment.

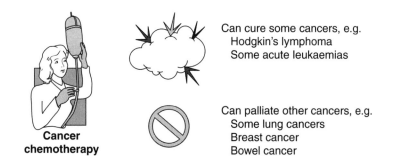

Can cure some cancers, e.g.
  Hodgkin's lymphoma
  Some acute leukaemias

Can palliate other cancers, e.g.
  Some lung cancers
  Breast cancer
  Bowel cancer

The drug regimes used depend on the type of cancer, the size of the patient and whether the aim of treatment is curative or palliative.

How can I use this information?

As cells die they are replaced by new cells. Cells divide at different rates and faster growing cells tend to be more sensitive to chemotherapy drugs. Some chemotherapy drugs also kill 'resting' cancer cells. Rapidly growing normal cells are also damaged (bone marrow, lining of the gastrointestinal and genitourinary tracts, ovaries, testes, skin and hair follicles).

How is cancer chemotherapy given?

Dose: the oncologist calculates the dose based on the patient's size, blood count, kidney and liver function.

Using drugs together: using several cancer chemotherapy drugs together kills more cancer cells, minimises the damage to normal cells, and reduces the chance of the tumour becoming resistant to treatment.

Divided doses: it is usual to give courses of treatments at intervals of 3–4 weeks. This is important as it gives normal cells time to recover before the next dose is given. Because cancer cells recover more slowly, the number of cancer cells steadily reduces. The number of courses varies; often 3–6 are planned. The final number depends on the response of the tumour and progress of the patient.

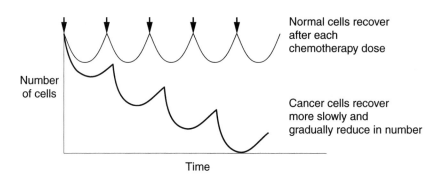

Getting chemotherapy into the body: only a few chemotherapy drugs are well absorbed by mouth. Most have to be given directly into the bloodstream, sometimes through a fine tube used long-term. Occasionally drugs can be given directly into the blood vessels supplying the tumour, or injected directly into spaces such as the abdomen, the spine or the space between the lung and chest wall.

Helping normal cells to recover: in some regimes other drugs are used to 'rescue' normal cells (e.g. folinic acid), or prevent them from being damaged (e.g. mesna to prevent cystitis). Removing the patient's bone marrow and then replacing it after treatment is another way of restoring normal cells.

Key points

- Many cancers respond to chemotherapy, but only a small number of types of cancer can be cured.
- The effects of chemotherapy are dependent on the dose, type and combination of drugs used.
- Most chemotherapy is given intravenously and on an outpatient basis.

Chemotherapy: side effects

What should I know?

Four points need to be remembered:

1 The differences between tumour cells and normal cells are small, so the balance between response (killing cancer cells) and toxicity (side effects) needs to be carefully considered.
2 Side effects depend on the drug and dose used.
3 Effective treatments keep side effects to a minimum – they are much less when the intention is palliation.
4 Some side effects are uncommon.

Tissue affected	Possible side effects of chemotherapy
General	Fatigue, loss of appetite
Skin	Loss of hair (not all chemotherapy drugs do this), dry skin
Feelings	Anxiety, low mood, fear
Mouth	Soreness, dryness, increased risk of infection such as yeast infection (thrush)
Bone marrow	Because bone marrow contains the blood producing mechanisms of the body there might be anaemia, bruising
Immune system	and perhaps bleeding because of too few platelets. Infection as a result of reduced numbers of white cells is a serious risk, especially 7–14 days after a dose has been given (occasionally delayed for 4–5 weeks)
Bowel	Nausea and vomiting (within a few hours or delayed for several days), diarrhoea
Kidneys	Reduced kidney function
Heart	Reduced heart muscle function
Lung	Breathlessness
Ovaries, testes	Infertility
Nerves	Reduced sensation, and feelings of pins and needles in the hands and feet

How can I use this information?

You might be involved in preparing a patient before receiving chemotherapy. You might observe some of the effects mentioned above and you may be involved in treating side effects or rehabilitating a patient following treatment.

Preparing the patient: it is important to be positive, as many side effects are temporary or can be effectively treated. The start of chemotherapy may be the first time a patient has had to face the reality of their condition.

Treating side effects: this may involve you in:

- giving drugs to stop any nausea, vomiting or diarrhoea
- ensuring the patient receives sufficient fluids
- keeping the mouth clean and moist, or treating a sore mouth

- being alert for signs of infection, especially fever, chills or shivers, since infection needs urgent medical attention
- watching for other side effects.

Supporting the patient: while some chemotherapy causes few problems for the patient, some regimes make people feel very ill and emotionally low. They will need understanding and the opportunity to express their feelings.

Key points

- The likelihood of side effects depends on the drug and doses used.
- Most of the effects of treatment are temporary and respond to treatment.
- Signs of infection are important to look out for as urgent medical attention is usually needed.

Hormone therapy

What should I know?

The growth of some cancers is dependent on natural hormones and some drugs reduce the levels of these natural hormones. If patients with hormone-dependent cancers are treated with these drugs, the growth of their cancers can be reduced or even stopped. Although cure is not usually possible, these drugs have been used with success to prevent a cancer that has been treated successfully with other treatments from returning (chemotherapy, surgery, radiotherapy or a combination).

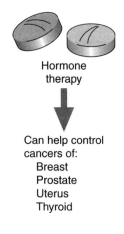

Hormone
therapy

↓

Can help control
cancers of:
Breast
Prostate
Uterus
Thyroid

What types of cancer can be helped?

Of the following cancers many, but not all, rely on natural hormones for their growth.

Breast cancer: 70–90% of these depend on oestrogen.
Prostate cancer: growth partly depends on testosterone.
Cancer of the uterus: 70–80% of these partly depend on oestrogen
Thyroid cancer: this depends on a hormone called TSH (thyroid stimulating hormone).

Examples of drugs used in hormone therapy

Drugs acting against oestrogen

- **Tamoxifen**
  Commonly used as the first choice in treatment, and often used to prevent return of the breast cancer after successful treatment.
- **Aminoglutethimide**
  Used if recurrence of breast cancer develops. Since it also reduces the body's natural steroids, replacement steroid (such as hydrocortisone) is also given.
- **Anastrazole**
  Acts like aminoglutethimide but steroid replacement is not needed.

Drugs acting against testosterone for prostate cancer

- **Cyproterone, flutamide**
  These are used as the first choice for treating prostate cancer.

Other drugs

- **Medroxyprogesterone, megestrol acetate**
  These are used to treat breast cancer and cancer of the uterus.

Side effects of hormone therapy

Most are well tolerated, but side effects do occur:

Drugs acting against oestrogen: hot flushes and altered monthly periods are the most common, but weight gain and dizziness can occur. Long-term use to prevent cancer recurrence may remove the protective effect of oestrogen in the body, causing an increased risk of osteoporosis and cancer of the uterus.

Drugs acting against testosterone: a reduced sex-drive is common with some drugs (cyproterone acetate) but is much less likely to occur with others (e.g. flutamide). They can cause breast enlargement in men but other side effects are unusual. Older drugs (e.g. diethylstilboestrol) are used less frequently because, although effective, they initially cause an increase in the growth of prostate cancer – called a 'tumour flare'.

Key points

- Some cancers (breast, prostate and uterus) depend on natural hormones for growth.
- Drugs that suppress these natural hormones can reduce or temporarily stop cancer growth.
- Not all cancers of the breast, prostate or uterus respond to this approach.

Section 3
Supportive and palliative care

- What is palliative care?
- Principles of palliative care
- Palliative care: who and when?

What is palliative care?

What should I know?

Palliative care has a specialist and a universal approach (supportive care). It is the universal approach that we will be concentrating upon throughout this book.

Throughout this book we will be supplying you with information and ideas for you to think about that will lead to you being comfortable with this approach.

Some definitions

To cloak or shield

The word *palliative* has its origin in the Latin verb *'palliere'* meaning to *'cloak'* or *'shield'*. Palliative care aims to provide support and enable patients to deal with distressing symptoms and the concerns they have associated with an advanced and progressive disease which cannot be cured.

A safe place to suffer

Working in a hospice in Oxford in 1987, Averil Stedeford gave us this definition of palliative care. At first it seems strange to include the word 'suffer', but what she meant was this:[1]

- however well you control the symptoms, some suffering is left
- it is helpful for patients to be able to talk about their distress

1   Stedeford A (1987) *Palliative Medicine.* **1**: 1–2.

- they will only talk if there are no distracting physical symptoms *and* they feel safe to talk
- helping people to feel 'safe to suffer' can be done in almost any setting (home, hospital or hospice).

An arc of care

Recently, David Roy, Director, Centre for Bioethics in Montreal wrote that:

> 'Palliative care arcs widely: rising where people hear the first foot falls of mortal illness nearing; landing and tarrying, there on the ground where the bereaved . . . weep, mourn and bury. An arc of care, an embrace gathering sureness over time.'[2]

Palliative care therefore:

- includes many conditions (not just cancer)
- starts at the time of diagnosis, but becomes increasingly needed (and more complex) as the illness advances
- can be done well in almost any setting.

How can I use this information?

It is important that you understand the difference between the universal palliative care (supportive care) and specialist approaches to palliative care.

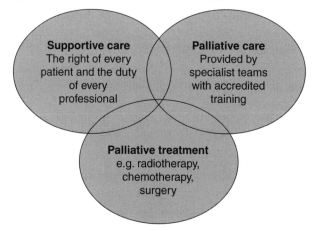

2   Roy D (2001) *Journal of Palliative Care.* **17**: 3–4.

Supportive care

This is the universal palliative care that everyone should be providing, regardless of the diagnosis, the discipline or the speciality. Supportive care is the right of every patient and the duty of every professional.

Palliative care

There are times when the problems are so complex that advice and supervision are required from doctors, nurses or other professionals who have recognised expertise and accreditation in palliative care. Specialist palliative care may be delivered directly when one or more professionals with specialist skills in palliative care will look after the patient for a period of time. Alternatively you may continue to deliver care and treatment according to the advice and subsequent review of specialist palliative care practitioners.

Palliative treatment

Sometimes patients may require surgery, radiotherapy, chemotherapy or some anaesthetic procedure. This additional treatment will not cure but will relieve a particular symptom. Although this is called palliative treatment, it is not the same as palliative care.

Key points

- No matter what your position in the organisation is, you have a role in the delivery of supportive and palliative care.
- The essence of supportive and palliative care is about being comfortable and confident that you have something to offer patients who are distressed or concerned as a consequence of advanced progressive disease.
- You are not alone – other team members have knowledge and skills that complement yours.

Principles of palliative care

What should I know?

No matter what the role you have in providing palliative care, you should aim to incorporate into your personal approach the following principles with patients, their close family and friends and with your colleagues.

- **Quality of life**: the best possible quality of life for patients – this includes good symptom relief.
- **Patient choice**: the preferred choices of the patient in relation to treatment options, future care and the place of care.
- **Open communication**: sensitive communication involving patients, their partner, family and all relevant professionals.
- **Whole person**: attention to the whole person taking into account past and present life circumstances.
- **Whole family**: care of people with the life-threatening disease and those who matter to them.
- **Whole team**: palliative care requires the skills of a group of different professionals working together, whether the patient is in hospital, at home or in a care home.

Principles of symptom control[1]

Effective palliative care is the right of every patient and partner, and the duty of every professional: access to training, updating, and to palliative care specialist services should be widely available.

Ensure adequate team skills, knowledge, attitudes and communication: individuals and teams need basic skills in communication and diagnosis, together with the knowledge of symptoms in advanced disease, their effects and management.

Create a 'safe place to suffer': this is not a building, but the relationship between carer and patient, one that enables the patient to feel safe to express their distress. Not all distress can be removed, but the expression of that distress is therapeutic.

Establish a partnership with the patient, the partner and family: the flow of information and treatment decisions should be controlled by the patient and negotiated with the partner and family.

Do not wait for a patient to complain – ask and observe: patients with persistent distress do not always look distressed. They may be withdrawn, with poor sleep or mobility, and the effects of the pain may have spilt over into the partner or relative. Assessing these factors is more important than estimating severity which is open to bias and often unhelpful in deciding treatment. The comments of the partner or relative are often helpful.

Accurately diagnose the cause of the problem. problems are often multiple and mixed. In advanced cancer, for example, 85% of patients have more than one site of pain, and 40% have four or more pains.

Treatment should be individualised: a successful choice requires a clear diagnosis together with the willingness to modify the choice depending on the response. This tailors the treatment to the patient.

Do not delay starting treatment: symptoms should be treated promptly since they become more difficult to treat the longer they are left. This is partly because their persistence makes it increasingly difficult for the patient to cope. In neuropathic pain, for example, the longer pain persists, the more pathways and

1 Regnard C and Hockley J (2002) *A Clinical Decision Guide to Symptom Relief in Palliative Care*. Radcliffe Medical Press, Oxford.

receptors are involved, making control much more difficult. Treatment must start as soon as the diagnosis is made.

Administer drugs regularly in doses titrated to each individual, that ensure the symptom does not return: if a drug gives effective relief for 4 hours, then prescribe it 4-hourly. 'As required' or 'p.r.n.' administration on its own will not control continuous symptoms.

Set realistic goals: first, accept the patient's goals. If these seem overly optimistic, negotiate some additional *shorter* term goals. If the patient's goals seem overly pessimistic then negotiate some additional *longer* term goals. A clear plan of action based on negotiated goals helps the patient and partner see a way out of their distress.

Re-assess repeatedly and regularly: accurate titration of medication demands reassessment.

Empathy, understanding, diversion and elevation of mood are essential adjuncts: drugs are only part of the overall management.

Principles of symtom control

- Patient's right, professional's duty.
- Adequate skills.
- Safe place to suffer.
- Partnership.
- Ask and observe.
- Diagnose accurately.
- Individual treatment.
- Do not delay.
- Regular medication.
- Realistic goals.
- Reassess.
- Feelings matter as much as drugs.

Key points

- Palliative care is about wholeness: whole patient, whole family and whole team.
- Patient choice is central, whether about information, treatment or place of care.
- Good symptom control relies on accurate diagnosis, realistic goals and titrated treatment.

Palliative care: who and when?

What should I know?

Everyone provides palliative care. Or at least, they should. Universal palliative care (supportive care) is the right of every patient and the duty of every professional. In many cases doctors and nurses will be able to deliver this care.

How can I use this information?

Occasionally, further help and advice ensures more effective palliative care. Consider seeking help in the following situations.

Unfamiliar situations

Diagnosis: a diagnosis that is uncommon in your practice may present new problems.

Symptoms: a symptom that is uncommon to you may have a simple solution you can obtain on discussing the problem with a specialist. Other symptoms may necessitate the patient being seen by a palliative care specialist.

Drugs: some symptoms in palliative care need drugs or routes of delivery that may be uncommon in your practice. Using resource texts, the internet or discussing the drug with a specialist may be all you need.

Persistent or severe symptoms

Physical or psychological problems can sometimes be difficult to resolve. If first- and second-line treatments have failed, discussion with, or a visit by, a palliative care specialist can offer new options.

Complex situations

Some patients have a complex mix of physical, psychological, social, ethical and spiritual issues which can make clear-cut decisions difficult. Discussion with a palliative care specialist can help you to see the situation more clearly.

Asking for help

- Unfamiliar situations.
- Persistent or severe symptoms.
- Complex situations.

Where can I ask for help?

Community palliative care team

They may give specialist advice, a one-off consultative visit or develop short-/long-term input. They work in close liaison with the general practitioner and district nurses. Community palliative care team support should be discussed with the general practitioner before the patient is discharged.

Hospice

St Christopher's Hospice Information Service (Tel: 020 778 9252 or www.hospice information.co.uk) publishes a directory of all hospice services in the UK.

Most hospices are mainly funded by local or national charities and provide specialist inpatient care. Patients have a range of diagnoses, including AIDS, progressive neurological disease, as well as cancer. There may be facilities for day hospice care, particularly valuable for patients who live alone or to enable the carer to have 'time out'. Some have outpatient facilities and a day treatment service. Specialist staff include specialist nurses, physiotherapists, occupational therapists, social workers, chaplain, counsellors and consultant physicians in palliative medicine who will see patients as outpatients and can also advise through ward or domiciliary visits. Such services offer telephone advice to all professionals (often 24 hours a day) and run active educational and research programmes.

Hospital support team

This is often initially Macmillan-funded and consists of specialist nurses and consultants in palliative medicine, with varying input from doctors, social workers, chaplains and physiotherapists. They are available to give advice and support to patients, families and staff in hospital and will liaise with community services.

Key points

- Everyone should be providing supportive care.
- Help may be needed in unfamiliar situations (diagnosis, symptoms or drugs), persistent or severe symptoms, or in complex situations.
- Help and advice will be given by palliative care teams in community, hospital or hospice.

Section 4
Cancer pain

- What is pain?
- What sorts of pain are there?
- When a patient is in pain, what should I do?
- Drugs used to treat pain
- Isn't morphine dangerous?
- What do I do if the pain is getting worse?

What is pain?

What should I know?

Here are three definitions. Which one best explains pain for you?

- Pain is perceived along a pathway that runs from pain receptors in tissues to the brain, and is modified at every step along its travel.
- Pain is an unpleasant, complex, physical and emotional experience.
- Pain is what the patient says it is.

The first definition sounds academic, while the last sounds simplistic. However, the last definition is the most helpful since only the patient can really know what their pain is really like. The second definition is a compromise between the two and might be preferred by those who prefer a 'proper' definition!

During their training most professionals meet patients with acute pain (e.g. a fracture) and are much less likely to meet a patient with chronic pain (e.g. neuralgia), let alone be taught how to manage such pains. So, if the patient's report of *'what pain is'* is not accepted, misunderstanding will result. Here are the important differences between acute and chronic pain.

	Acute pain (e.g. fracture)	Chronic pain (e.g. neuralgia)
Patient	Obviously in pain	May only seem depressed
	Complains loudly of pain	May only complain of discomfort
	Understands pain	May see pain as unending and meaningless
	Primarily affects the patient	Pain overflows to affect family and carers
Carer	Treatment is straightforward	Treatment may be complex
	Injected analgesics OK	Analgesics by mouth are preferable
	Analgesic side effects acceptable	Analgesic side effects unacceptable

How can I use this information?

In one recent survey, 88% of patients with advanced disease had pain in the last year of life and 66% found this pain 'very distressing'.

So in practice you can expect around 60% of patients with advanced disease to get troublesome pain. Interestingly, this figure is similar for AIDS, heart disease and disorders of the central nervous system.

Pain may remain for many reasons. Here are some of the reasons, with their consequences (you may have thought of some more).

Reasons	Consequences
Belief that pain is inevitable	Unnecessary pain
Inaccurate diagnosis of the cause	Inappropriate treatment
Lack of understanding of analgesics	Use of the wrong analgesics, wrong dose or not given regularly
Unrealistic objectives	Dissatisfaction with treatment
Infrequent review	Rejection of treatment by patient
Lack of attention to mood and morale	Increased sensitivity to pain

Key points

- Pain is what the patient says it is.
- Most causes of unrelieved pain are unrelated to analgesics.
- Chronic pain cannot be treated the same as acute pain.

What sorts of pain are there?

What should I know?

Only tissues and structures containing pain receptors can cause pain. There are only a few tissues that have these receptors – muscle, skin and nerves are the main ones.

Brain tissue, bone marrow, blood and liver tissue do not have pain receptors to cause pain. Some structures only have pain receptors in their outer coverings – bone and liver are two examples.

The number of possible causes of pain is even more limited. Injury, local pressure, inflammation, infection, loss of blood supply, and nerve damage are the main causes.

Neuropathic pain is a special type of pain that does not need pain receptors. Neuropathic pain includes pains such as neuralgia in the face due to trigeminal nerve damage, or the neuralgia that can develop after *Herpes zoster* (shingles) infection. Any nerve damage can cause changes in the spinal cord and brain. This can make unpleasant, painful sensations persist even though no pain receptors are involved.

How can I use this information?

Being clear about what can cause pain and the different structures involved will help you to work out what causes of pain might be associated with some everyday activities as set out in the first table on p. 62.

Types of pain

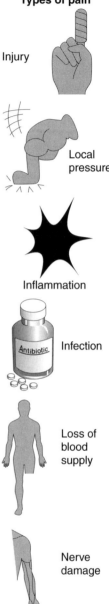

Action causing pain	Possible cause of pain
Eating	Sore mouth, gullet or stomach
Worsened by the slightest passive movement	Bone fracture
Straining a bone	Bone damage causing weakness
Contracting muscle against resistance	Muscle pain or strain
Moving a joint	Arthritis
Taking a deep breath	Pleurisy
Sitting down	Pressure sore over sacrum

'*But*' you might think '*what about pain that is not brought about by specific action*'.

You then need to take account of how the pain is '*behaving*'. Some common characteristics of pain are listed in the table below.

Characteristic	Possible cause of pain
Coming and going every few minutes	Colic, e.g. constipation
Red skin	Local skin damage, e.g. pressure sore
Unpleasant sensory change at rest	Neuropathic pain, e.g. shingles neuralgia
Pain felt in an area supplied by a peripheral nerve	Nerve pressure or damage, e.g. sciatica

These characteristics are important observations that form the basis for diagnosing pain. So it is important that you report exactly what the patient tells you and any other observations that you make that will help the clinical team make accurate decisions about treating pain.

Key points

- Despite the many pain syndromes, there are only a few causes of pain.
- Pain usually involves tissues containing pain receptors, the exception is neuropathic pain.
- Understanding the different characteristics of pain is the basis for diagnosing pain.

When a patient is in pain, what should I do?

What should I know?

Start by believing what they are saying!

It is very rare for patients to imagine they have pain, and usually they are very consistent in how they describe their pain. Some patients may not be able to say they are in pain, but they looked distressed, and you, the partner or family suspects that the patient is in pain.

Severe pain and distress

If the pain is obviously very severe and the patient is very distressed you need to report this immediately to the nurse or doctor responsible for the patient's care.

Breakthrough pain

The pain you are witnessing might be breakthrough pain. This can happen when the patient's pain is being closely monitored and regular analgesia has been prescribed. Some change may have happened to alter the dose requirement of the analgesic that the patient is regularly taking, so if you have the authority and have had instructions about giving analgesia for breakthrough pain then go ahead and give what has been prescribed.

Check for simple causes

Next, you should find out more about the pain so check for simple causes, for example:

- has the patient slipped into an uncomfortable position?
- is something on the chair or in the bed making them uncomfortable?
- has the patient missed his regular medication?
- does the pain suggest colic that might indicate constipation?

How can I use this information?

You have established that the patient has pain and you are aware that you need to report this. Sometimes as a carer you can feel let down because you think that the information you passed on has been ignored. It may be that you haven't given sufficient information for the doctor or nurse responsible for the patient's care to appreciate the importance of what you have reported. You can do a number of things to strengthen your message.

First, make the patient as comfortable as you can. Then find out more about the pain. For example:

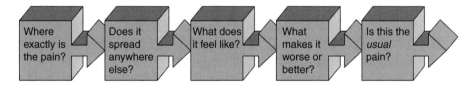

Some more points

- It is a good idea to write down the details as the patient is telling you. The patient then knows that someone is paying attention to the pain.
- If you have the authority, write these details in the patient's record sheets. If not, you should still write them down on separate paper and pass them on to the nurse or doctor who is looking after the patient.
- Sometimes it can be helpful if you or the patient draw the pattern of the pain on a diagram of the body. This is useful when the patient has several different pains.

- Some teams use pain severity scales. Although these do not help in diagnosing or treating the pain, they can be used to convince sceptical colleagues about your patient's pain!
- Finally, it is useful to know if the patient is anxious, frightened or low in mood. These emotions will make it more difficult for the patient to cope with their pain and can be a cause of persistent pain.
- The pain may be preventing the patient from carrying out their favourite activities such as gardening or walking. See if you can make these activities less painful, e.g. using a wheelchair.

Key points

- Pain is what the patient says it is.
- If the pain is severe get some analgesia or get help.
- Check for simple causes.
- Find out about how the pain is affecting the patient.
- Always write the information down to ensure that the appropriate person takes action.

Drugs used to treat pain

What should I know?

Drugs that treat pain are known as analgesics. It would be very simple if all analgesics relieved all types of pain. Unfortunately life is never that simple!

Some analgesics work directly on a pain (such as paracetamol for headache). Opioids are the largest group of direct analgesics used in palliative care and examples are weak opioids, such as codeine, and strong opioids, such as morphine.

Other drugs work indirectly. For example, an antibiotic will stop the pain caused by infection. These indirect analgesics are known as adjuvant analgesics and they are used for different pains.

Directly acting analgesics	Indirectly acting analgesics (adjuvants)

Non-opioids
  e.g. paracetamol, nefopam
	To treat neuralgia
	Low dose antidepressants
	  e.g. amitriptyline
	Anticonvulsants
	  e.g. carbamazepine

Opioids
Weak opioid
  e.g. codeine
Strong opioid
  e.g. morphine
	To reduce swelling
	Corticosteroids
	  e.g. dexamethasone

Non-steroidal anti-inflammatory drugs (NSAIDs)
  e.g. ibuprofen
	To reduce muscle spasm
	Antispasmodics
	  e.g. hyoscine butylbromide
	Antispastics
	  e.g. baclofen

Nitrous oxide 1:1 with oxygen (e.g. Entonox)	*To treat infection* Antibiotics e.g. amoxycillin

Principles of using analgesics

Doctors use three well-established principles when prescribing analgesics:

By the clock

Giving the analgesic regularly gives continuous pain relief.

By the ladder

Low doses of weak analgesics are gradually increased and then changed to stronger analgesics. These adjustments are known as titration and allow analgesics to be adjusted to each individual.

By the mouth

Patients prefer to take analgesics by mouth rather than by injection or suppository.

How can I use this information?

A basic understanding of analgesics can help you explain to a patient or relative why a drug regime has been changed. A universal guide for prescribing analgesics is the World Health Organization (WHO) analgesic staircase which uses non-opioids, weak opioids and strong opioids, with the option to use adjuvant analgesics at any stage.

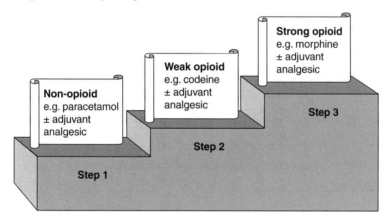

Creating an individualised analgesic staircase

The standard 'analgesic staircase' only applies to pain that responds to opioids like morphine or codeine. In reality, pain can have many causes, and several pains can co-exist, sometimes in the same site. Each patient therefore needs an individualised analgesic staircase.

In severe pain in cancer, we usually start with opioids since several pains are often present together and one of these is commonly opioid-sensitive. However for skin pressure pain, the staircase would be very different. In addition, if a person is anxious, this too needs to be included in the staircase along with any other emotional or social issues. Acknowledging such needs is essential to help the patient cope more effectively with pain.

Therefore, a staircase for an anxious patient with a painful pressure sore might look like this:

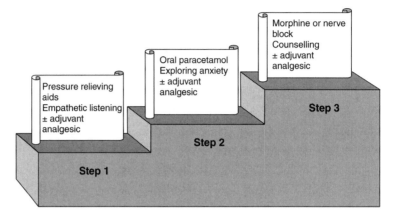

Step 1
Pressure relieving aids
Empathetic listening
± adjuvant analgesic

Step 2
Oral paracetamol
Exploring anxiety
± adjuvant analgesic

Step 3
Morphine or nerve block
Counselling
± adjuvant analgesic

Key points

- Different analgesics work with different pains.
- Some analgesics work through secondary mechanisms.
- Different pains may need different analgesics.

Isn't morphine dangerous?

What should I know?

Patients and carers have a number of concerns about morphine:

- **Will I get addicted?**   No.

You may have thought this did not matter since it is more important to treat the pain but addiction would be an added insult to an already complicated situation, especially for the many patients who live for years with their illness. In reality it is rare to see addiction in patients who take morphine for cancer pain.

- **Will it wear off?**   No.

Even after months or years, doses of morphine do not have to be increased if the disease is stable. If the illness gets worse then doses may have to be increased, but evidence shows that the longer a patient is on morphine the more likely they are to *reduce* the dose or *stop* the morphine altogether! The reason for this is that another drug or treatment may be added to help control the pain.

- **Will I get drugged?**

One of the useful features of morphine is that if drowsiness occurs, this wears off within a week in most patients. Many patients can safely drive their cars once their dose is stable. The fact that drowsiness wears off quickly makes morphine a useless sedative and it should never be used to try and 'settle' a patient or make a patient sleepy.

• **What about other side effects?**

A dry mouth is common. About one-third can feel sick or vomit, but this is controllable with other medicines, and wears off after 1–2 weeks. Confusion due to morphine is uncommon, unless the dose has been increased too quickly – most confusion in advanced disease has other causes. Some patients have vivid dreams on morphine, but hallucinations are rare. Since many side effects of morphine wear off, morphine is always started at low doses and gradually increased, often avoiding side effects altogether. So breathing problems are not seen in patients whose dose is low to start with and gradually increased. Constipation is inevitable and a regular laxative is needed to prevent it occurring.

• **Does it mean the end?**   No.

Morphine is now started whenever needed. The decision to use morphine has nothing to do with the severity or stage of the illness. It is about being pain free. Many patients take morphine for pain other than cancer pain.

• **Does morphine kill you (or do you die sooner)?**   No.

There is no evidence that morphine shortens life when it is used correctly. Doctors and nurses in hospital, community and hospices can, and do, use morphine correctly without problems. The doses are adjusted to the patient's pain, and the right drugs are used to help the specific problem. Used correctly, morphine is safer than many drugs available in the high street pharmacist.

• **Can you be allergic to morphine?**   No.

There are cases of getting an itchy rash with morphine, but this is rare when using morphine to treat pain.

• **Can everyone tolerate morphine?**

Most people tolerate it well. Some people do not tolerate morphine because of persistent drowsiness or confusion. Sometimes this is because they are sensitive to its effects, or on other occasions poor kidney function allows some of the by-products of morphine to build up. This is not a problem, however, as these patients can be changed to other analgesics that are just as effective as morphine.

How can I use this information?

This information should be used to ease the fears of patients, relatives and members of staff who are new to seeing morphine used for pain.

Key points

- Addiction is not seen in patient's taking morphine for pain control.
- Pain relief due to morphine does not wear off.
- Many side effects of morphine do wear off. Constipation is an exception and is treated with laxatives.
- Used correctly, morphine does not kill patients.
- Most patients can tolerate morphine, but alternatives to morphine are widely available.

What do I do if the pain is getting worse?

What should I know?

When pain persists despite treatment everyone gets disheartened. Staff sometimes feel they have let the patient down and the patient begins to feel that they will never get rid of their pain. This makes some patients angry, frightened or emotionally low – problems which can make it more difficult for them to cope with their pain. So a vicious circle begins that may lead staff to start avoiding the patient and cause the patient to become increasingly distressed.

How can I use this information?

Remember pain is what the patient says it is – so you will want to explore the pain. Pain can persist for many reasons.

A simple checklist can help.

1 **Is the diagnosis of the pain correct?**
   This is the time to reassess the pain. New information should be reported to those who are managing the pain.
2 **Are the analgesics appropriate?**
   For example, there is no point in using morphine to treat colic since it may make the colic worse.
3 **Is this a new pain?**
   New pains can appear, and it is easy to assume that the old pain is persisting.

4 **Is the patient taking the drugs correctly?**
Patients may not be able to take oral medication because they are feeling nauseated, or may refuse to take the medication.

5 **Has an indirect (adjuvant) analgesic been used?**
These are drugs which treat pain indirectly.

6 **Have other treatment options been considered?**
Radiotherapy is effective in treating 80% of cancer deposits that have spread to bone, often with single treatments given as an outpatient. Rapid and long-term pain relief can follow surgery to put a metal pin in a leg bone weakened by cancer. Massage and relaxation can help reduce a patient's anxiety.

7 **Is the patient anxious, frightened, agitated or depressed?**
Many issues can complicate pain, for example advancing disease, low self-esteem, unfinished business, or the memory and experience of a friend or relative who died from cancer. Even in the face of eventual death, hope is important, but this can be affected in many ways.

Factors that influence hope in the terminally ill	
Increased hope	*Decreased hope*
Feeling valued	Feeling devalued
Meaningful relationship(s)	Abandonment and isolation
Reminiscence	Conspiracy of silence
Humour	There is nothing more to be done
Realistic goals	Lack of direction or goals
Effective pain and symptom relief	Unrelieved pain and discomfort

It may seem strange to suggest keeping up hope in these situations, but it is fairly easy to do. A patient can be helped to shift from hope of cure, to hope of attending a wedding, or hope in maintaining independence and comfort. Of course, if it is clear that depression is present, this needs treatment. (See *Fostering hope*, pp. 161–3.)

8 **Have you asked your local pain or palliative care team?**
If the pain is still a problem, ask for help!

Key points

- When pain persists, reassess.
- Run through the persistent pain checklist.
- Look out for underlying anger, fear or depression.

Section 5
Symptoms

- How can I help a patient who is constipated?
- What can I do when a patient is nauseated or vomiting?
- How can I help a breathless patient?
- How can I help a patient with fatigue and weakness?
- What can I do when a patient does not want to eat or drink?
- Maintaining an environment for eating
- How can I help a patient with mouth problems?

How can I help a patient who is constipated?

What should I know?

This might seem easy. Most people would feel that going less often than usual means they are constipated. This idea works fine if you are eating normal amounts, drinking normally, and fully active. But this is unlikely to be the case for people with advanced disease. It is normal for these patients to pass stools less often. So we need to use other definitions.

Patients tell us that they feel a number of sensations when they are constipated:

- an uncomfortable or painful stool
- fullness, despite opening their bowels
- abdominal colic (a pain in the abdomen that comes and goes every few minutes)
- opening their bowels less often
- diarrhoea (caused if the stool is causing a bowel blockage)
- nausea (a feeling of queasiness)
- loss of appetite.

Of these, the first two (discomfort and fullness) are the most useful. This means that a patient passing a comfortable stool every 6 days is *not* constipated. It's a question of *quality not quantity*!

Causes of constipation

When you realise that a stool becomes hard because it is drier than usual, it becomes easier to think of causes. Several causes will make a stool lose water.

Not drinking enough: this makes a patient thirsty and causes more water to be absorbed from the bowel.

Slowing the bowel: this makes the stool stay longer in the large bowel so that it loses more water. There are many causes of slowing the bowel, such as drugs (e.g. morphine), being less active and depression.

Eating less fibre: this has two effects:

• the bowel is less active, so the stool stays longer in the bowel, becoming drier and harder
• the stool is less able to hold on to water.

How can I use this information?

The best treatment is to prevent it happening in the first place!

Prevention

1   Help the patient understand what is meant by constipation.
2   Keep a record of the quality of bowel motions.
3   Make sure a patient is drinking enough fluids.
4   Start laxatives at the same time as drugs that cause constipation (e.g. morphine).
5   Help a patient to be active and eat what they can, although this will become more difficult for them as they become more ill.

Treatment

Is this a bowel blockage? One possible cause of producing no stool at all is a blockage of the bowel (this may be due to cancer) or to the bowel being paralysed (some drugs can cause this 'ileus'). Although both are much less common than constipation, the doctors looking after the patient must exclude these as a possible cause.

Laxatives: these are often necessary in patients with advanced disease, especially if they are taking constipating drugs such as morphine. A combination of stimulant and softener has been found to be most useful in advanced disease, especially if patients are on analgesics such as codeine or morphine.

- *Stimulants*: these make the bowel contract harder than usual, so the stool moves through faster with less time to dry out. Most act only on the large bowel, e.g. senna.
- *Softeners*: these are either concentrated syrups, e.g. lactulose, which acts by drawing in water from the bowel wall making the stool wetter, or laxatives which prevent the stool from drying out, e.g. docusate.

Enemas: these are last resorts because prevention was not done or was unsuccessful. They are not a treatment for constipation. Either oil is used to lubricate the stool, or a stimulant solution is used to make the bowel contract.

Key points

- Constipation is defined as an uncomfortable stool accompanied by a continuing sensation of fullness.
- The main causes are constipating drugs, reduced fluid and fibre intake and reduced activity.
- Prevention is the key – monitoring regularly and starting laxatives early are essential.
- Enemas are a last resort, not a treatment.

How can I help a patient who is nauseated or vomiting?

What should I know?

Nausea and vomiting affects nearly two-thirds of patients with advanced cancer. Both are very distressing when they persist.

The causes of nausea and vomiting

Psychological: anxiety and fear can cause nausea and vomiting or make them worse.

Chemicals: there is an area in the brain, which continuously checks for troublesome chemicals in the blood and the fluid around the brain. Some chemicals cause this area to stimulate nausea and vomiting. For example:

- chemicals from bacteria or the environment
- drugs used to treat symptoms, e.g. morphine for pain
- drugs used to treat cancer (chemotherapy drugs)
- chemicals produced within the body, e.g. too much calcium.

Problems with emptying the stomach: drugs can slow the emptying and cause food and drink to build up in the stomach until the patient produces a large vomit, perhaps only once a day. Nausea is brief, occurring just before the vomit, with the patient feeling more comfortable after they have vomited. Occasionally, the exit of the stomach is blocked and this causes forceful vomiting and makes the patient lose fluids quickly over one or two days.

Irritated stomach: drugs and anxiety can both cause the lining of the stomach to become inflamed causing a 'gastritis'. In severe cases this can progress to an ulcer.

Other causes: there are other important causes whose mechanisms are not clearly understood, for example:

- bowel distension
- constipation
- cancer in the chest or abdomen
- increased pressure inside the skull due to cancer.

How can I use this information?

Having an awareness of the range of causes of nausea and vomiting helps you to be on the alert and reduce the fear and embarrassment that often accompanies this symptom. When a patient vomits you should:

- find a large bowl (or bucket) and a towel; small bowls simply guarantee that the vomit will end up all over the bed!
- hold or sponge their forehead (whichever they find most comforting).

Treatment of nausea and vomiting

Treatment will depend on the cause. This might be soothing an irritated stomach, helping to reduce anxiety, treating an infection or correcting abnormally high blood calcium. On many occasions it is necessary to use a drug to stop the nausea and vomiting.

These drugs are called antiemetics and they work in different ways:

Help empty the stomach: these help the stomach empty more normally, preventing the build up of food and fluid, e.g. metoclopramide (Maxalon).

Treat chemical causes: these act on a set of receptors in the chemical sampling area of the brain, e.g. haloperidol (Serenace).

Used during chemotherapy: these are effective in treating nausea and vomiting due to chemotherapy, but have very little use in other types, e.g. ondansetron (Zofran).

With a broad action: the antiemetics above have specific actions. Sometimes the type and cause of the nausea and vomiting are unclear. In this case the use of a 'broad action' antiemetic is useful, e.g. cyclizine (Valoid) or levomepromazine (Nozinan).

When one antiemetic is insufficient, two are sometimes used in combination.

Key points

- Remember a large bowl and towel first.
- The most common causes are a poorly emptying stomach, an irritated stomach, chemicals and anxiety.
- Treat the cause if possible.
- Select antiemetics according to the cause – sometimes two antiemetics together are more effective.

How can I help a breathless patient?

What should I know?

Breathlessness is as common as pain in cancer, but is often more frightening and disabling. Unless the cause can be treated, simple measures are often the most important.

Telling if breathlessness is present

- Patient complains of breathlessness on moving. When severe the patient may be breathless when talking or at rest.
- The patient looks 'out of breath'.
- Finger nails or lips have a blue colour. A blue colour to the fingernails or lips happens if the amount of oxygen in the blood is low. However, some patients can have low oxygen levels and yet look pink – they need to be checked with a simple machine that shines a light through a fingertip (an oximeter).
- Confusion or agitation may accompany the breathlessness.
- Anxiety is common in a breathless patient.

How quickly did breathlessness start?

Sudden breathlessness, starting in seconds or minutes, has different causes (e.g. a blood clot to the lungs) from breathlessness that builds up over days or longer (e.g. a growing cancer).

How can I use this information?

Reporting any of the signs accompanying breathlessness will alert the doctor to examine the chest and carry out other investigations such as a chest X-ray. These will help to decide what is causing the breathlessness.

Simple measures

Cool air: the simplest action is to increase the movement of air over the patient's face using a fan or opening a window. This has been shown to make patients feel less breathless.

Help the patient to sit upright: this makes breathing easier by allowing gravity to help pull down the diaphragm.

Encourage the patient to relax the shoulders: breathlessness is frightening and one of the effects of fear is to tense the shoulders. This reduces the amount of air getting into the lungs. Concentrating on relaxing the shoulders makes breathing easier.
  Try it yourself:
- tense up your shoulders and take a deep breath
- relax your shoulders and take a deep breath
- easier with relaxed shoulders, isn't it?

Massage the shoulders: this will help them to relax. Standing behind or to one side of the patient means the patient only has to concentrate on your voice and touch. Partners and families can be taught easily to do this massage.

Distraction: encourage the patient to seek company, a television, radio or music to help distract them from the breathlessness.

Explain: don't forget to explain what you are doing and, if you know, why the patient is more breathless.

Other treatments

Oxygen: a trial is worth trying. There is no reason to worry about the patient becoming 'hooked' on their oxygen. Nasal cannulae are better tolerated than a mask. In the home or in some of the voluntary hospices the source initially will be an oxygen cylinder, but an oxygen concentrator can be prescribed if oxygen is going to be used for 15 hours or more each day.

Drugs: steroids may reduce swelling around the lung tumours to free up more normal lung tissue for taking up oxygen. Low doses of morphine and tranquillisers can ease breathlessness when it is troublesome.

Acupuncture has been used with some benefit.

Breathlessness clinics: some patients have benefited from breathing retraining and breathlessness clinics are beginning to be established.

Severe breathlessness

Agitation most often accompanies severe breathlessness. The key is to manage the agitation, which is probably being caused by the low oxygen levels in the blood. If none of the previous measures have helped, and the patient is distressed, then the a low dose of a sedative is helpful. Some sedatives relax rather than cause drowsiness and can be taken in tablet form. Others are more sedating and can be given as a continuous injection under the skin from a small portable pump.

The key to helping such patients is to use the lowest dose that settles the patient with as little drowsiness as possible.

Key points

- Breathlessness is common and distressing for the patient.
- Simple measures can be the most effective.
- Drugs are of limited help, except in severe breathlessness.

How can I help a patient with fatigue and weakness?

What should I know?

Drowsiness, tiredness, lethargy, loss of strength, fatigue and weakness can all have different meanings for different patients. For one patient it might mean weakness or a lack of energy; another patient might describe a loss of strength. There are three useful definitions:

Drowsiness: a sensation of sleepiness and difficulty staying awake.

Loss of strength: having insufficient power to carry out an action due to paralysis or loss of muscle.

Fatigue: a sensation of tiredness or having insufficient energy to carry out activities.

How can I use this information?

Thinking about the three above definitions might help you to understand the causes of these distressing symptoms:

Drowsiness: might develop rapidly, gradually or slowly.

- Rapid drowsiness occurring over hours or days suggests a cause that might be related to drugs, breathing, infection or chemical imbalances in the blood (e.g. high calcium).
- Gradual drowsiness increasing over weeks could be due to liver damage, gradual accumulation of long-acting drugs or poor quality sleep (causing daytime drowsiness).
- Slow drowsiness developing over months might be due to the effects of a cancer or loss of sleep due to anxiety or depression.

Loss of strength: this may be localised or generalised.

- Localised loss of strength can be due to nerve damage, or damage to a part of the brain as in a stroke. In some cases, the loss of strength is localised to the shoulders and hips and this can be caused by a range of problems such as steroids or a low potassium level in the blood.
- Generalised loss of strength is seen when muscle is lost due to inactivity. It is also seen in cancer, infection or severe heart problems as part of a process called *'cachexia'*. This process is 'switched on' by the cancer or infection and results in muscle being broken down into unwanted energy. Up to three-quarters of muscle can be lost in this way.

Fatigue: has many causes including infection, insufficient food, depression, anaemia and treatments such as surgery, radiotherapy and chemotherapy. Fatigue is also an important part of the process of *'cachexia'*. Fatigue is not due to a cancer or infection competing for energy with the body.

Simple measures for fatigue and weakness

It is essential to treat the cause if this is possible. In the meantime, or while waiting for treatment to work, simple measures might help.

Treat other symptoms: make sure that other symptoms such as pain, nausea and vomiting have been treated, since persistent, severe symptoms are themselves exhausting.

Prepare the patient for a good night's sleep: avoid tea and coffee in the evenings (suggest milk or alcohol instead). Check for low mood and anxiety and if present inform team members experienced in assessing and treating mood problems. A sleeping tablet might help.

Modify the activities that cause fatigue:

- use rest periods between activities
- plan regular gentle exercise and arrange help for activities that are a low priority for the patient
- re-time activities to a time of day when the patient feels they have the most energy.

Key points

- Patients use many different words to describe different aspects of this problem.
- Drowsiness, loss of strength and fatigue are the most useful definitions to use.
- The cause should be treated, but if this is not possible then it is possible to modify activities so they cause less fatigue.

What can I do when a patient does not want to eat or drink?

What should I know?

As activity diminishes in the last weeks of life it is normal to eat less, and in the last days and hours of life, it is normal to drink less. It can be difficult to decide how much food and drink is appropriate at any particular time.

Assessing the situation

These questions will help you and the patient to decide what is needed:

1 **Is the patient deteriorating day by day because of the illness?**
   If it is clear that the deterioration is due to the illness (and not to something that is easily treated), then this suggests time is becoming very short. There is no right or wrong decision about food and drink at this time.
   At this stage, food and drink can no longer keep someone alive, but may provide essential comfort and pleasure. What the patient and partner together feel is best for them is your most useful guide.
2 **Are there reasons why appetite is reduced?**
   This is known as anorexia. Some causes, listed below, are treatable:

- pain
- fear or depression
- constipation
- nausea and vomiting
- breathlessness
- infection
- odour
- drugs, e.g. chemotherapy.

Other causes cannot be treated at present. In some patients the cancer changes how the body uses energy causing anorexia and loss of fat and muscle. This is called cachexia and is a very different process to starvation (tumours use up less than 5% of the body's energy needs).

3 **Is feeding or drinking difficult?**
Check for difficulty in swallowing, or that the patient is not too weak, breathless or disabled to be able to eat by themselves.

4 **What is the food like?**
At this time patients find large portions unappetising. This might upset people at home who are trying hard to maintain normality. It is important to make sure that the patient is in a comfortable eating position. A little thought can make food appear much more appetising. Be sure to help if the patient is unable to remove covers, or is having difficulty using cutlery or cutting the food into small portions.

5 **Does the patient want to eat?**
Patients may feel they do not wish to eat any more. This is not a problem if depression has been excluded, and everything has been done to improve food presentation and appetite.

How can I use this information?

There are many ways of helping. Start with simple measures.

- Keep the mouth moist with water sprays and cool drinks.
- Keep portions to small, attractive snacks. Vary the taste, consistency and temperature.
- Avoid unpleasant smells and cooking odours with ventilation and avoid strong perfumes.
- Make sure any food is correct for the patient's culture, e.g. kosher food.
- Give the patient privacy to eat if they are embarrassed about eating.
- Help the patient to eat and drink if they are unable to do so themselves.

- Causes of a reduced appetite need to be treated, and swallowing problems assessed and treated if possible.
- Food supplements (as drinks or powder) can be helpful, especially cold, but they need to be taken in small amounts through the day. Supplements tend to be poorly tolerated when taken all at once.

Despite trying to help, many patients still have a problem with appetite. This can be part of the cachexia syndrome, which also causes fatigue and weakness. In cachexia the cancer does not 'use up' energy needed by the body, but instead the body changes some of its chemical processes into ones that waste energy. As yet, there is no specific treatment for cachexia. Steroids have been used with some improvement in appetite, although they can cause problems if used over a long time.

Key points

- If time is very short, eating and drinking might be solely a comfort and pleasure.
- Treat causes of a reduced appetite.
- Simple measures are often the most effective.
- Steroids help some patients for a short while.

Maintaining an environment for eating

What should I know?

We eat for many reasons:

- nutrition
- hunger
- survival
- habit
- boredom
- choice
- pleasure
- social activity
- satisfaction
- comfort.

Many things influences our choice of diet:

- likes/dislikes
- religion
- resources (e.g. money)
- budget
- occasion
- environment
- medications
- illness, loss of taste
- physical/mental health problems.

Above all, eating should be a pleasurable activity.

How can I use this information?

This can have a big impact on a person's wish to eat or take part in mealtimes.

On the whole we can choose when we eat, what we eat, where we eat and with whom. Having this choice allows eating to be a pleasurable and social activity and not just a means of survival.

For some, this means eating in the company of others. However, other people prefer privacy, especially if they already have difficulty eating.

Problems with the mealtime environment

Timing: daily routines in places like hospitals and nursing homes can lead to inflexible mealtimes with limited time allocated for serving, eating and enjoying a meal.

Size of area and number of people: a crowded small room is not conducive to pleasant mealtimes, nor is a large area with open access or thoroughfare. Thought needs to be given to the number of people using the dining room.

Unintentional exclusion: positioning of the patient, carer and furniture needs to be carefully thought out to prevent unintentional exclusion, for example a patient facing a blank wall, but hearing general activity behind them.

Presentation of food: each meal should offer variety, be attractive, be the correct temperature and appropriate portion size for the patient.

Equipment: if necessary the patient should be assessed by an appropriate professional (i.e. physiotherapist, occupational therapist) for seating and use of crockery/utensils. Otherwise the usual furniture needs to be checked for table height and access.

Communication: this is an extremely important part of eating so distractions and background noise, for example music, stacking plates, should be kept to a minimum. Relationships should be acknowledged both between patients and between patients and staff and, wherever possible, the patient's choice should be exercised.

Communication opportunities increase for both the patient and carer when the carer pays attention, is responsive, is at face-to-face level, gives eye contact, asks simple questions, creates choices, uses simple language about the meal, and allows the patient to use all sensory information, for example sight, smell, touch.

Lessons to be learned

1 The dining area should balance space and sociability.
2 If it is necessary to feed someone the carer should sit opposite the person being fed, and talk calmly providing verbal and non-verbal prompts and encouragement.
3 Appropriate sized mouthfuls should be given with time allowed to enjoy the meal.
4 Food should be colourful and well seasoned so it stimulates the appetite via sight, smell and taste.
5 Portion size should be individually adjusted and consideration given to the individual needs of the patient and to the temperature of the food offered.
6 Many people assume that anyone can assist another to eat. However, feeding a patient is not a simple procedure. Carers need to be taught how to do it, what the problems are and how they might be overcome. Most importantly, they need to know the danger of choking.

Key points

- Eating is a pleasurable, social activity as well as being essential for health.
- Problems with mealtime include inflexible routines, poor dining facilities, unattractive food, insufficient help and forgetting about encouraging communication.
- Assisted feeding is a skill that requires training.

How can I help a patient with mouth problems?

What should I know?

We breathe, eat and speak through our mouths. So it is essential that our mouths are clean, moist, pain-free and able to hold food and fluids. Patients with advanced disease often get oral problems and to prevent these problems it is necessary to:

- brush teeth or dentures twice daily with toothpaste containing fluoride
- keep mouth moist by ensuring good oral fluid intake.

There is a range of problems that palliative care patients might experience.

The patient may have difficulty holding food and fluids in the mouth: a local cancer, or damage to the nerves controlling the muscles of the tongue or cheeks will cause difficulty with swallowing. Such patients present a high risk of having a dirty mouth.

A dirty mouth: this may simply be debris on the teeth, gums or tongue. White patches suggest an infection called 'thrush', caused by a build up of yeast called *Candida*. This needs to be treated.

A dry mouth: anxiety causes a dry mouth as do some drugs and infections. However, it may be that the patient is not drinking enough fluids.

A painful mouth: there might be a mouth ulcer (apthous ulcer), or pain could indicate infection, local cancer or damage to the sensory nerves of the mouth. A common cause of pain is badly fitting dentures.

How can I use this information?

It is important to encourage patients and/or their carers to regularly examine the mouth and teeth. However, you may be the carer and have the opportunity on a day-to-day basis to undertake this important task.

When inspecting the mouth look at the tongue, lips, gums, throat, the roof of the mouth and inside the cheeks. Start with the simple things.

- Ask the patient about dryness or pain and check their mouth regularly for any sign of ulcers or debris.
- Make sure the patient is drinking enough fluids to prevent thirst.
- Make sure the patient is brushing their teeth or dentures twice daily with toothpaste containing fluoride. Check that dentures are a good fit.
- For a dry mouth, keep the patient supplied with cool, non-alcoholic drinks. Simple sprays of water also help.
- For a dirty mouth, clean the teeth and rinse the mouth regularly. Chewing tinned, unsweetened pineapple may also help.

If you discover something is wrong, you need to let other members of the team know since various actions need to be considered.

- Infections need to be treated.
- Encouraging the patient to drink an increased amount of fluid may remedy a shortage of body fluid or the situation might require giving fluids through a vein or under the skin.
- Difficulty in swallowing may need to be investigated to find the cause.
- If drugs are causing a dry mouth, the dose will need to be changed or a different drug used.
- If pain is a problem, pain-relieving mouthwashes or gels will need to be prescribed; occasionally, stronger drugs have to be used.

Key points

- Prevention is important and includes regular brushing of teeth and inspection of the mouth.
- Simple measures are helpful and need to be continued.
- Other team members will be needed if the problems persist.

Section 6
Communication

- Why is communication so important?
- What can I do to relieve a person's anxiety?
- How do I answer a difficult question?
- What about breaking bad or difficult news?
- How can I help an angry person?
- How can I help a withdrawn patient?
- How can I help a confused patient?
- Do children understand what is going on?
- How does illness affect how we see ourselves?
- Identifying distress when communication is poor

Why is communication so important?

What should I know?

What is communication? Communication is our way of letting each other know who we are, what we know, and how we feel about ourselves, other people and the world around us.

It's not just words. Although we usually communicate by talking, it is the way we act and look that gives meaning to the words. We tend to respond to our own interpretation of what someone is saying to us. This means that communication is affected by the circumstances and relationships between the people communicating. It is a matter of how messages are perceived. Because this process is complex and automatic it is possible for us to respond to a situation without knowing or understanding our behaviour.

What affects communication? Not surprisingly, many things can affect communication, such as deafness, speech distortion, pain, depression, tiredness.

How can I use this information?

1   It helps us to appreciate why simple words can create different responses in different people.
2   It explains why listening is the key.

Listening

Listening is hard work!

To listen well to ill and distressed people you have to:

- remove distraction, e.g. choose a quiet comfortable room with chosen company
- reduce misunderstanding by asking the person to clarify the words and feelings they expressed, e.g. 'Can you explain what you mean when you said you lie awake worrying at night?'
- explore any thoughts or feelings that are troubling them, e.g. 'What sort of things make you feel anxious?'

Listening also means that you are a receiver as well as a sender of information. This means you need to be aware of how different messages affect you. Your own experiences might affect how you appear to the other person. This need not deter you from entering into communication with others. You just need to be aware of how you are feeling and that you might confuse your own experience with the other person's feelings.

For example, you might be tempted to say, 'I know exactly how you feel, my father had the same problem.' However, it is the other person's feelings you are checking, not your own! So, saying something like, 'Can I check what you are saying and feeling at this moment?' can help to ensure that you are receiving the messages correctly.

Approaching listening in this way is an active process, not simply passively soaking up the words! For this reason, it is called 'active listening'.

Support for you

It is wise always to seek support for yourself when you are frequently involved in communication with other people about distressing events or feelings. Most healthcare professionals have a system of practice supervision or clinical supervision in place to help staff reflect on how they deal with this type of situation.

Key points

- Communication is not just words, but an interaction between two people.
- Effective listening means removing distractions, and reducing misunderstanding by clarifying words and feelings.
- Try to avoid confusing your own feelings and experiences with those of the other person.
- Seek support if you are often involved in communication with others about distressing events or feelings.

What can I do to relieve a person's anxiety?

What should I know?

People are usually clear in saying if they feel anxious, worried or frightened. Some people try to hide their anxiety but it will tend to show in other ways, such as irritability, anger, poor concentration, tiredness or lack of sleep. It is very difficult for people to hide all their anxiety and most anxious people will look or feel apprehensive, tense or on edge. On rare occasions, a very frightened person looks 'frozen' with fear. These people look pale, with dilated pupils and a fast heart rate, and may need urgent help with their fear.

Certain drugs might be the cause, for example anxiety states can happen if drugs given to treat insomnia, anxiety and depression have been suddenly stopped. Other drugs can cause restlessness and fidgeting. This can make some people look anxious, but they will soon tell you the problem is restlessness, not anxiety.

How can I use this information?

1 **Acknowledge the anxiety**: as with many situations where emotions are involved, acknowledgement of the anxiety or fear shows you noticed and that you care. This may only mean saying something like, 'You seem worried today'.

2 **Touch**: touch is a valuable mode of communication but you need to be sure that this is acceptable to the person. Gentle touch communicates the message of sharing the fear. Some people will withdraw from touch – this can be a sign that they need to remain in control.

3 **Explore the reason for the anxiety**: this indicates that you want to help. It may be possible at this stage to provide what the person needs, such as company, help or information.

4 **Relaxation and distraction**: introducing some relaxation and distraction techniques might lessen anxiety associated with the ongoing circumstances that are likely to persist:
- distraction: company, radio, television, CDs or tapes to reduce time spent feeling anxious
- relaxation: music, massage, peaceful places can all do this. People can be taught relaxation exercises, which they can use when they are alone
- massage: some patients will accept simple massage (e.g. on the neck or shoulders) or aromatherapy with relaxing oils.

5 **Sleep**: anxious people require the assurance of a good night's sleep: a peaceful environment helps as does a bedtime drink – milk or alcohol are best (but avoid a late evening tea or coffee). Sleeping tablets are a last resort.

What do I do if the person is still anxious?

If these simple measures don't reduce the anxiety, then more professional help is indicated. This might be found within the regular team or outside specialist help may be needed. If a person is agitated, tormented, very disorganised or 'frozen', urgent help is needed.

Examples of some situations that require more help follow.

- **Anxiety state**: this is present when:
  - anxiety is present for more than half the time for more than 2 weeks
  - it is different from their usual mood
  - four or more anxiety features are present such as fear, irritability, poor concentration, restlessness, and sweating.
- **Poor function**: troublesome anxiety will reduce concentration, but if the anxiety is severe enough, people may be unable to care for themselves or make a decision.
- **Panic attacks** are common in troublesome or severe anxiety. They occur suddenly without an obvious cause, are intense and can last 5–20 minutes. A fear of dying or losing control is often part of these episodes.

- **Phobias** are situations or objects when help is impossible, difficult or embarrassing. These require specialist intervention to enable the person to avoid the cause.
- **Frozen terror**: a person can be so frightened by their situation that they are 'frozen', unable to move or speak. However, the body's automatic response to fear will continue to be active, i.e. you will be able to detect dilated pupils, a fast heart rate, pallor and sweating.

Key points

- Anxious people appear apprehensive, tense or on edge.
- Start by acknowledging the fear, with gentle touch, asking what's wrong and providing simple help.
- Further help is given by using distraction, relaxation, massage and ensuring a good night's sleep.
- Additional help will be needed for persistent or troublesome anxiety, panic, phobias or frozen terror.

How do I answer a difficult question?

What should I know?

Patients, partners and relatives may ask you a question which you find difficult to answer.

- **Surprise**: often the question is asked when you least expect it, adding to its difficulty.
- **The patient, partner and relative**: they require information to make rational choices, but this may conflict with the fears of advancing illness and the need to maintain hope in the face of uncertainty. These conflicts often result in difficult questions.
- **For the professional**: there are fears of admitting ignorance, being blamed, producing an emotional reaction, or of dealing with a situation for which they have received little or no training. These make questions more difficult to answer.
- **Setting**: because difficult questions are often spontaneous, the setting may be awkward, such as a busy corridor. It is reasonable to offer a quieter location if the person asking the question wants this.

How do I use this information?

1 **Acknowledge the importance of the question**. It usually takes the person much thought, anxiety and courage to ask the question. This needs to be recognised, e.g. 'That's an important question'.

2 **Find out why the question is being asked**. This avoids any misunderstanding. You could ask something like 'I wonder why you're asking me this now?'

Case example:
At the end of a morning clinic, a patient asked the doctor 'How much longer have I got?' The doctor asked the patient why he had asked that question, only to find that the patient wanted to know whether the interview would finish in time for lunch!

Checking gives the person an opportunity to make sure how willing they are to hear the answer.

3 **Are you the right person?** You need to consider if you are the most appropriate person to be answering the question. If the answer is straightforward, clear and you are comfortable in answering, then provide the answer.

4 **If the person seems reluctant to hear the answer**, check the following:
- you need to be satisfied that the person is not troubled with drowsiness, deafness or confusion

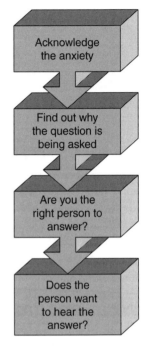

- check that the person wasn't put off because you weren't paying full attention! The most likely reason is because the question caught you unprepared. You can remedy this easily by apologising for the inattention and once more acknowledge the importance of the question
- the person may suspect that any answer is going to be bad or difficult news. (See *What about breaking bad or difficult news?*, pp. 110–13.)

Is the answer still difficult?

There are good reasons why you may be unable to answer the question:

- inexperience
- you don't have the information the person needs
- it's an emotionally charged question (e.g. 'Am I dying?').

You need to be honest with how you feel:

'I don't have the experience (or knowledge) to answer that question, but I'll get someone who can.'
'I'm finding that difficult to answer.'
'I don't know what to say.'

People will respect your honesty, which demonstrates that you are taking their question seriously. It will be reassuring for the person to know that you will not abandon them so offer a future contact time:

> 'I'll be interested to hear how you get on with . . . If you want to talk about it with me later please do.'

Some questions don't have simple answers – be honest and admit you don't know.

There are some questions that have no clear answer because full information is not available. An example would be the patient who asks when they are going to die. Again, being honest with the situation is helpful. Start by acknowledging the uncertainty:

> 'I can see this uncertainty is difficult for you.'

You will be able to see if the person can accept small chunks of reality such as what they understand about their illness, for example:

> 'How does it look to you at the moment?'

If you think the answer will be bad news then once again you need to be prepared to ensure that an appropriate person can take the communication further. (See *What about breaking bad or difficult news?*, pp. 110–13.)

Key points

- Questions can be difficult because of conflicts in the patient, partner or professional.
- Start by acknowledging the importance of the question and asking why they have asked the question.
- Being honest about your reaction to a difficult question is important and often appreciated by the person asking the question.

What about breaking bad or difficult news?

What should I know

Bad news is bad – you can't make it less bad! People with experience in breaking bad news will tell you that it is an uncomfortable and sometimes distressing task. Inevitably the information is sad and will draw on the emotional strength of the recipient who might be a patient or a relative. In reality you cannot assume that news is bad or good, it's impact depends on whether the person will find it difficult to take on board.

Good practice involves:

- finding somewhere quiet and private to talk
- letting the person be in control of the situation, i.e. asking for permission in the first instance to talk about the subject, then allowing the person to take the lead about the nature, quantity and depth of information being discussed
- being prepared for silence
- encouraging reflection on small chunks of information and giving clarification
- avoiding jargon – if some slips out, re-phrase it in the person's words.

How can I use this information?

Three things to check

1 **The person's understanding**: this involves making sure that the person can hear and is capable of understanding. Confusion, anxiety and depression can all reduce concentration.
2 **The person's knowledge**: this is crucial. It is wrong to assume. For example, the doctor might ask, 'What have you understood about the tests so far'?
3 **The person's desire to know more**: this is not as difficult as it sounds. For example, 'Do you want me to explain the results of the tests?'

Nearly all patients and relatives have some advanced warning that something might be wrong, e.g. a biopsy of a suspicious lump. In most cases, there is the opportunity to ask them what more they want to know. It is rare that people have absolutely no idea that any bad news is on the way.

Check the person's:

1 Understanding.
2 Knowledge.
3 Desire to know more.

Three reactions people could have

1 More information is requested – 'I think it's better that I know'.
2 No more information is wanted – 'Oh, I'll leave all that to you'.
3 Uncertainty about how much information is wanted – 'I'm not sure'.

If the person is uncertain, the carer might ask some further questions:

'Are you the sort of person who likes to know everything that is happening to them?'

If the uncertainty persists this is best acknowledged and left open. The carer might say:

'I can see you're not sure. That's not a problem, you can ask me sometime in the future'.

This does not prevent the discussion of treatment. This may seem strange but remember that someone is unsure about knowing more because they are struggling to cope with the truth. Discussing treatment is a way of getting on with things and helps them to cope.

Possible reactions:

1 More.
2 Stop.
3 Unsure.

The three step approach:
WPC (Warn, Pause, Check)

Most people are already worried that something might be seriously wrong. Even so they still need to be warned that this is the case. The Warn/Pause/Check approach is used. A typical discussion might be:

1 **Warn**
  Carer: 'I'm afraid the results were more serious than we thought.'
2 **Pause** – wait for a response.
  Person: 'What do you mean more serious?'
  Carer: 'We found some abnormal cells.'
3 **Check**
  Carer: 'Do you want me to explain what these were?'

It is important to check that the person has understood the news. This WPC approach is repeated until the person has all the information they want at that time. It is equally important that the person knows that 'the door is open' to return for further information or clarification. It is good practice to offer a follow-up interview.

WPC approach

1 Warn.
2 Pause . . .
3 Check.

Three final checks

1 **Acknowledge any distress**: for example, 'I can see how you're feeling about this'. People worry most about the emotional reaction of a person being told bad news. Whether or not the person is accepting the bad news, there are likely to be elements of anger, anxiety and depression, hidden or overtly displayed. A reaction is normal. You might be with someone soon after bad news has been given. It is important to acknowledge that you know this has happened. Ask something like, 'How are you feeling?'

2 **Is the person overwhelmingly distressed?** Don't underestimate the value that your presence and your acknowledgement has for a person at this time. Time is needed to absorb bad news. You may not have to do anything more than 'be there'.

3 **Is the person denying or holding unrealistic expectations?** If a person chooses not to believe what is happening (denial) this needs to be accepted as a normal coping mechanism. This should only be challenged if it is clear the person remains distressed and is not coping – this must be left to someone skilled in helping such patients. On the other hand you might find that you could help a person articulate feelings and perhaps questions that can be answered by more experienced staff.

Final checks

1 Acknowledge distress.
2 Is distress severe?
3 Is the person unrealistic?

Key points

- Bad news is always difficult – you can't make the news less bad, but you can avoid breaking it badly!
- The professional's task is to find out how much the person wants to know, rather than to decide what to tell.
- Use the WPC method: Warn, Pause, Check – this allows the patient or relative to control the rate of information.
- It is normal for a person to react emotionally after being told bad news.

How can I help an angry person?

What should I know?

Anger is a very natural response to fear or to feeling wronged. Usually the anger is obvious, but sometimes people try to hide their anger. Most people are affected emotionally when confronted by an angry person.

- Some will feel irritated, while a few will react by becoming angry themselves.
- Others do the opposite and will draw back, while a few become very passive in the face of anger.

It is important to check which of these feelings you have when you are met with anger. If you are someone who becomes angry when facing anger, then ask someone more composed to deal with the situation. If you are someone who becomes very passive, then ask someone who can be more assertive in the face of anger.

> Check how anger affects you.

You need feel no embarrassment in withdrawing from a situation involving anger. It may be that you are tired or feeling stressed at that moment. It is better to withdraw than to risk inflaming a situation. On another occasion you might be more composed (or more assertive) and able to respond. If on the other hand you believe that you lack the appropriate skills, then make this known to your manager who can arrange for you to have appropriate skills training.

How can I use this information?

1 **Acknowledge obvious anger**: knowing that anger is a natural response should enable you to acknowledge what is going on: 'I can see you are angry. How can I help?'

2 **Check for hidden anger**: if you suspect that the person is controlling his/her anger, you may have to start by saying, 'I get the feeling that you're angry, how can I help?' and wait for their response.

3 **Setting**: you can suggest an appropriate setting to deal with the situation but it's usually impossible to choose the right setting. If the setting seems particularly awkward (e.g. a busy corridor) then as the discussion progresses it is reasonable to suggest an alternative venue.

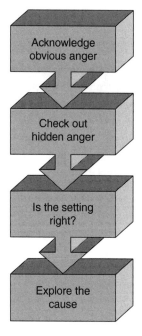

4 **Exploring the anger**: as soon as you acknowledge the anger it should begin to subside. Anger is often a response to frustration, so offering to help is important. The help may be with action or giving information. Exploring the cause of the anger in itself helps to defuse it since this draws attention to the needs of the angry person. Try to discuss the cause, for example, 'What has caused you to feel angry?' Often anger is justified in that:

- its reasons can be understood
- it is understandable that some people in distressing situations become angry.

When to apologise (and when not to)

When the anger is directed at you, and that anger is appropriate then come clean and apologise! 'I'm sorry you were kept waiting for so long – it would make me angry too.'

When the anger is about the behaviour of another health professional, avoid the temptation to defend that person since:

- it's not your place to defend others
- trying to defend the other person will fail to defuse the anger.

You can still show your concern without being defensive, 'I can see why you're angry, I think I would be too'.

Escalating anger

Your actions so far should have reduced most people's anger within minutes. At the very least, it should be no worse. Occasionally, however, the anger escalates. *This is an important warning sign.*

- Acknowledge the escalating anger. 'I can see that you are still angry.'
- Move to the door.
- From the door, set limits for continuing. 'It's difficult to continue whilst you're so angry and it's important that we resolve this today – can you control your anger so that we can continue?'
- If the person cannot accept the limits, offer another time to discuss the situation and *leave the room.* Failure to leave the room increases the risk that you are attacked.
- If the person accepts the limits, continue the discussion but stay by the door until it is clear the anger is lessening.

Persisting anger

You need to consider some of the reasons why people are persistently angry. There are times when people need specialist help through counselling. Persistent anger can accompany clinical depression, spiritual unrest, a strong reaction to the consequences of the illness, unfulfilled ambitions, such as it not being possible to see children grow up, or frustration through loss of control because of weakness or immobility.

Key points

- Start by checking how you are feeling and if you are sufficiently composed to deal with the situation.
- Acknowledge the anger and offer to help.
- Check how appropriate the anger is.
- You can apologise for your mistake, but never apologise for someone else's!
- Beware of escalating anger since there is a risk of violence.

How can I help a withdrawn patient?

What should I know?

There are many possible reasons why a patient could be withdrawn:

- perhaps by nature the person is reserved
- speech and facial expressions may be severely affected by conditions such as motor neurone disease, Parkinson's disease or drugs that can reduce movement as a side effect
- pain, anger or anxiety may be so severe that it is preventing them from concentrating
- a confusional state may be making them suspicious or unwilling to talk
- drowsiness caused by drugs or chemical disturbances in the blood may be preventing a conversation
- the patient may be reluctant to talk for fear of upsetting a partner or relative
- they may be too exhausted to talk, or they might be too frightened to talk (the 'frozen terror' syndrome)
- they may be suffering from depression.

Depression

It has been suggested that 25% of patients with cancer and AIDS suffer from depression. The diagnosis of depression is made on the following features:

- there is a persistent low mood (more than 2 weeks for more than half of the time)
- this is a change to their usual mood
- it is difficult or impossible to distract them out of their low mood
- four or more depressive-related symptoms are present, e.g. waking early in the morning, feeling worse in the evening, undue guilt, loss of interest in activities.

How can I use this information?

1 Check for understanding. The patient may be deaf or distracted by a confusional state. If the patient is deaf, check for a faulty or misplaced hearing aid. You could position yourself so that the patient can lip read without difficulty or you may have to find an interpreter of sign language, or use a mechanical or electronic speech communicator.
2 Treat any pain or confusional state.
3 Reduce drugs that may be causing drowsiness or side effects causing withdrawal.
4 Manage anxiety or anger.
5 Explore feelings such as embarrassment. The withdrawal may be due to a problem such as incontinence.

Your role

Your role is to notice and acknowledge what is happening. A helpful approach might be: 'You don't seem your usual self today', or 'Can you manage to tell me why you're finding it so difficult to talk?'

Treating depression

If a clinical depression is present, the doctor will prescribe an antidepressant. You are not likely to see a response to medication immediately. This can take up to 2 weeks. Treatment may be strengthened with therapy such as cognitive therapy which gives the patient skills that reduce the chance of the depression returning.

Sometimes the patient is the last to notice any improvement so your continued interest and support is very necessary. If the depression is persisting or has complicating features (e.g. agitation, paranoia) the doctor will seek advice from a psychiatric colleague.

Key points

- Acknowledge that the patient is withdrawn.
- Look for possible causes, depression is only one of many.
- If depression is present, an antidepressant is usually needed.
- Depressed patients may take up to 2 weeks to feel an improvement.

How can I help a confused patient?

What should I know?

Because confusion is an unfamiliar experience it is frightening and distressing. This is as true for patients as it is for those caring for them. Confusion has three main causes:

Altered brain function can be caused by problems such as drugs, infection, and chemical changes in the blood. These are the most common causes of confusion in advanced disease.

Distraction: a number of problems, if severe enough, can distract a patient to the extent that they function in a disorganised way. Examples are pain, anxiety and depression.

Brain damage may be due to dementia (a steady loss of brain cells over months and years), a stroke (either a bleed or loss of blood supply) or by a tumour (either starting in the brain or spread from a tumour elsewhere). A tumour is an uncommon cause of confusion.

What is confusion like?

It might be helpful to consider what confusion is like for the patient. Imagine coming in on Monday and all your colleagues tell you it's Tuesday. At first you laugh it off as a joke, but as they persist, you start getting angry with them. As the day wears on and everyone still insists it's Tuesday you start to feel anxious, wondering why they have picked on you. It doesn't take long before you start to feel frightened, wondering how you could have missed a whole day.

Most patients with confusion:

- have difficulty remembering recent events, names or people
- have difficulty concentrating
- have difficulty knowing the time and the place they are in
- have difficulty interpreting what is happening around them
- are frightened at what is happening and some may believe they are going mad.

There are two sorts of confusion:

Acute confusion

This is most commonly due to infection, drugs or abnormal blood chemistry. Its features are:

- it develops rapidly over hours or days
- a change in alertness (more drowsy or more alert)
- a change in severity from hour to hour.

Chronic confusion

Examples are senile dementia and the dementia associated with Down's syndrome. Its features are:

- it develops slowly over months or years
- there is no change in alertness
- there is little change in severity from hour to hour.

How can I use this information?

The first thing to keep in mind is that the patient is not going mad. They can still process information correctly, but the information they are getting has been 'filtered' by the cause of the confusion, causing them to make inappropriate decisions. So you can begin with making their environment more stable and giving them 'hooks onto which they can hang their reality'. For example:

- ensure there is a light, quiet and consistent environment (in hospital or hospice, this might be best in a single room)
- reduce the number of staff and visitors, but not the number of visits; they need the comfort of familiar faces
- on each visit remind them of who you are, where they are and what time it is
- keep all staff informed about progress or deterioration.

Problems needing extra help

The cause of the confusion must be searched for if possible and treated, but some problems will need more help and advice.

- **When the cause of the confusion is unclear**: morphine and brain tumours are often blamed, but these are uncommon causes of confusion.
- **If behaviour has altered**: this may cause the patient to feel suspicious of others (paranoia), excessively enthusiastic (euphoria or mania) or very low in mood.
- **If the patient is hallucinating**: this may be something the patient sees or hears, when there is nothing to see or hear.
- **If the patient is very agitated**.

Key points

- Confusion is frightening and confusing for patients, carers, visitors and staff.
- The commonest cause is drugs, infection and chemical changes in the blood.
- A light, quiet environment, a minimum of staff changes and gentle reminders of time and place will help.
- Further help is needed when the cause is unclear, behaviour has altered, the patient is hallucinating or the patient is very agitated.

Do children understand what is going on?

What should I know?

Although children's understanding of death varies with age, honest explanations and allowing children to talk about their feelings are important regardless of age.

Very young children understand the meaning of separation from a parent, but they may be unable to understand the permanence of death and may think that a parent who has died will return. This can cause profound grief. Pre-school children may be bewildered or appear to ignore death. Five to eight-year-olds are in the stage of 'magical thinking', believing that wishing can make something come true. They often become especially good and conscientious, as if in hope of restoring the dead. Older children express sorrow as adults do – they may be apathetic, withdrawn, cry a great deal or become hostile and angry.

Difficulties in coping with a parent's or grandparent's terminal illness are not always related to age, as older children are sometimes more withdrawn and uncommunicative than their younger siblings. Children need particularly sensitive understanding to help them cope with their awareness of the terminal illness and impending bereavement. Their needs for support should be explored.

A child's response to death can depend on what they have seen and learned from their family. The attitudes to death, openness with children and support they receive from the extended family can be important influences. Many couples do not talk to their children about the illness unless the children ask questions. Problems may arise in their bereavement if children are not involved when a close relative is terminally ill.

Examples of good practice

Anne (aged 7): she regularly visited her great grandmother in a nursing home. Over a period of time she witnessed the old lady becoming very frail. Her mother described great-gran's life as a flower, one that blooms, withers and dies. She encouraged continued contact through touch and kisses. Anne was visiting on the evening that great-gran died and asked if she could watch television. Mum and gran were sitting at the bedside. When the old lady died Anne continued to watch television for a short time, then cautiously approached the foot of bed, stood for a moment then returned to her television programme. A few moments later she returned and approached more closely. Without any prompts she moved in closely to her great-gran, kissed her and said goodbye. She turned to her mummy and said, 'Granny will sleep forever now'.

John (aged 4): his grandfather was very interested in John and spent time chatting to him about all sorts of topics. When the grandfather became terminally ill, John asked his grandfather if he was going to die. The grandfather told him that although he was going away, he would always look after him from a place far away where he wouldn't be able to see him. He told John that in this far off place he would be happy and able to walk again. When his grandfather eventually died John wanted to see him in his coffin. He wanted to check that grandfather had his shoes on. On the day of the funeral it was raining and John remarked that 'Grandad was dancing on the clouds'.

How can I use this information?

1 **Protecting or isolating?**: sometimes children are discouraged from visiting because relatives feel that it would be a strain or an embarrassment for the dying patient or because they feel that the children could be upset by what they may see. Although understandable, protecting children in this way risks isolating them with their own fears and imagination. While patients' and relatives' wishes must be respected, they may appreciate an opportunity to discuss their feelings with staff.

2 **Talking to children**: as with adults, it is helpful for one or two members of staff to introduce themselves by name and build trust with the child. Joining them in play is an ideal opportunity to get to know a child while allowing the adults time together. There are occasions when parents would appreciate advice about a child who is withdrawn or seems anxious, or they might seek

advice about whether a child should continue to visit when the patient's condition deteriorates. Staff may be able to support younger children by just talking to their parents or grandparents and encouraging openness within the family. Teenagers in particular may appreciate talking to a nurse or doctor alone.

3   **Facilities** such as a coffee lounge, a play area, or crèche may help children to feel more at home when visiting a relative in hospital or a hospice. Fostering an attitude among staff that recognises the distinctive relationships that exist between each member of the family and the patient, should be a key objective of care.

Key points

- Children's understanding of death varies with age.
- Children need particularly sensitive understanding to help them cope with their awareness of the terminal illness and impending bereavement.
- We should take time to speak to children and teenagers individually, as well as to adult family members.

How does illness affect how we see ourselves?

What should I know?

Self-image is a person's own impression of their physical appearance, and what sort of person they feel they are, something which may or may not be accurate. This image is built up from observing ourselves, the reactions of others, and a complex interaction of attitudes, emotions, memories, fantasies and experiences, only some of which we are aware of.

How does self-image develop?

From an early age we learn about who we are from the way that other people respond to us. Love, touch and the way our parents and family react to us is our first indication of being loved, liked, disliked, pretty, charming, difficult or clumsy. The more often such descriptions are made the more likely they will become part of our beliefs about ourselves. Social interactions affect body image through an individual's entire life.

As we grow older the same is true from the different interactions that we continue to have with people. This is like having a 'social mirror' in front of us, but unlike an ordinary mirror this is one that affects us deeply.

What sorts of self-image are there?

There are many parts to self-image:

- body image – how we see our bodies, e.g. thin, fat, handsome, ugly
- feeling image – what sort of person we think we are, e.g. kind, tough
- social image – how we feel we relate to other people
- sexual image – how attractive or repulsive we feel sexually
- achievement image – how we feel we have achieved our goals in life
- job image – our feelings of worth at work
- spiritual and ethical image – whether we see ourselves as good or bad people.

How does illness change self-image?

Appearance: if our body is damaged by cancer (e.g. a cancer affecting the face) or altered by surgery (e.g. mastectomy) this will deeply affect one's sense of self. After all, it is through our body that we express who we are to the outside world. These changes can alter our view of our body (body image), attractiveness (sexual image) and how we relate to others (social image).

Feelings: it is easy for serious illness to change the way we think about ourselves. We may believe that the changes of illness have changed the way we are (feeling image, social image) and we may blame ourselves for what has happened (spiritual and ethical image). This may show itself as anger (social image), depression or anxiety (feeling image).

Familiarity: illness calls for major adjustments to life and makes much of our lives unfamiliar because of attending hospital, visits from healthcare professionals and the reaction of others around us. A sense of isolation (social image) and a loss of self-worth can occur (achievement image, job image).

Threat: serious illness is a threat to our present and future life and symptoms such as pain or loss of function can be a constant reminder of that threat. This may stop us from setting goals (achievement image) and affect our self-worth at work (job image).

Function: physical illness and its treatment can reduce our ability to move or reduce our energy. This inevitably affects our body image, sexual image, achievement image and job image.

How can I use this information?

- Fostering hope and encouraging spirituality are important parts of helping someone with an altered self-image.
  Action: See *Fostering hope*, pp. 161–3 and *What is spirituality?*, pp. 164–6.
- A loss of self-image is about a loss of self-worth.
  Action: showing you are prepared to care for, and be with, that person demonstrates that you think they *are* worthwhile.
- Illness can make people feel they are 'dirty' or repulsive.
  Action: if the person agrees, touch can help. This may simply be a light touch on an arm, or the person may agree to try massage, aromatherapy or reflexology from a trained person.
- Many problems in illness such as odour, loss of function, pain or nausea can be treated or helped.
  Action: make sure the right people are involved, e.g. physiotherapist, occupational therapist, palliative care team.
- Psychological problems such as depression and fear can be helped.
  Action: make sure the right people are involved – the local palliative care team is a good first step.

---

1 Foster hope and encourage spirituality.
2 Be prepared to show that you think they are worthwhile, even if they don't.
3 Make sure the right people are involved.

Key points
- The feelings we have about ourselves are influenced by the reactions of other people.
- Self-image is made up of body, feelings, sexuality, social issues, goals, job worth, spirituality and ethical issues.
- Serious illness has profound effects on self-image.
- Help for altered self-image includes fostering hope, encouraging spirituality and treating symptoms, but the most important is to show you think that they are worthwhile.

Identifying distress when communication is poor

What should I know?

Patients have difficulty communicating in different contexts:

Coma: this is common in a patient dying of advanced cancer in the last hours or days before death. It can make it difficult to know if a patient is still distressed.

Cancer: primary or secondary tumours of the brain can cause difficulties.

Psychiatric conditions such as severe depression or psychosis will hinder or prevent communication and any acute confusional state will also hinder communication.

In addition, people with dementia or a learning disability can develop cancer, especially as improved care means that many are living much longer than before, e.g. 80% of people with Down's syndrome are aged 50 or over.

Brain damage: if this causes a severe drop in the ability to learn then communication is severely affected. The most common cause in children is a brain infection (encephalopathy) and in adults it is dementia. Shortage of oxygen at birth can cause cerebral palsy which in some children (but not all) causes difficulties in speech or understanding. Trauma or strokes can do the same.

Genetics: the most common is Down's syndrome, but only a minority are so severely affected that they have difficulty with communication. Other types cause rare chemical disorders which damage the brain.

Behaviours and signs of distress (the 'language' of distress)

There are many ways that people could express distress.

Sounds: these may be using language (simple descriptions, e.g. 'I'm not right'; associated words, e.g. always using the words 'My knee hurts' for any type of pain), or using sounds (crying, screaming, sighing, moaning, grunting).

Facial expression: these may be simple expressions (grimacing, clenched teeth, shut eyes, wide open eyes, frowning, biting lower lip) or more complex (where patients look sad, angry or in pain).

Easing the discomfort: rubbing or holding the area, keeping the area still, approaching staff, avoiding stimulation, reduced or absent function (reduced movement, lying or sitting).

Distraction: rocking (or other rhythmic movements), pacing, biting hand or lip, gesturing, clenched fists.

Posture: increased muscle tension (extension or flexion), altered posture, flinching, head in hands, limping, pulling cover or clothes over head, knees drawn up.

Automatic: there may be changes in the pulse rate, pupil size, skin colour or sweating.

How can you identify distress?

As with any language, you have to:

- know what the words mean
- learn a basic vocabulary
- know how the words are put together
- make sense of what the person is saying.

In people using alternative communication, the language is made up mainly of behaviours, signs and verbal expressions. The difficulty is knowing what these behaviours, signs and expressions mean (i.e. it's *us* who have difficulty understanding the person). They can only be understood with close observation. For example:

Nausea: this tends to cause an autonomic response with pallor, cold sweating and a slow pulse.

Fear: increased pulse, dilated pupils, tremor and increased respiration.

Frustration: crying or screaming, rapid and purposeless movements, looking angry.

Leg pain: holding the leg still, rubbing the leg, limping, refusing to move.

How can I use this information?

A real difficulty is that any cause of distress can be accompanied by any behaviour, sign or expression. We therefore need more information.

Is this behaviour or sign new?: for this we need to know their usual behaviour by recording baseline behaviour and asking the main or previous carers what they know.

Is this behaviour or sign associated with known distress?: for this we need to identify behaviours and signs with specific distress (e.g. during an episode of constipation or in a frightening situation). This can only be done if behaviour, signs and expressions are regularly documented.

If there is any uncertainty: local palliative care and learning disability teams can help – ask them.

Is the sign or behaviour new?

Document in detail signs and behaviours of distress.

If uncertain, ask for help.

Key points
- The language of distress consists of behaviours, signs and expressions.
- Documentation of distress signs and behaviours is essential if each individual is to be understood.
- The problem is *our* understanding.
- If unsure ask for help.

Section 7
Dying and bereavement

- What is loss and grief?
- How can I support the patient, partner and relative?
- How do I help with a dying patient's distress?
- What do I do when a patient dies?
- Death of a patient's friend or relative
- Supporting staff after a patient has died
- Complicated grief

What is loss and grief?

What should I know?

When someone has a life-threatening illness such as advanced cancer, thoughts about loss are common. For a patient these may be thoughts about loss of health, function, comfort or future life, while for a partner or relative it will be loss of the patient, and death and bereavement.

The 'loss' is felt early, often at the time of diagnosis, so the practical and emotional consequences need to be dealt with early on. These issues of loss are important in palliative care. The focus of interest is understandably on the person who is ill, but sadly, there is often inadequate attention given to the needs of the key people who will be left behind.

It is important first to look at the words that are used in the language around death – loss, grief, bereavement and mourning.

Loss

These are the feelings we have when we lose someone or something important. The experience depends on what a person regards as important in life. This might be relationships with family, friends, with people in general and sometimes pets. It might be health, riches, or the person's beliefs. All of these will have a different effect but what is clear is that loss is a constant part of our life, from infancy to our own death.

Bereavement

This is the term used to define the loss we feel following the death of a person or pet. Bereavement usually evokes similar and more powerful responses than other types of loss.

Mourning

This is the public face of grief. It is a social behaviour, which is moulded by experience and tradition, and is often very different from one culture to another.

Grief

This describes the feelings of bereavement. It involves physical symptoms and distortions of thought and emotions. Grief has a beginning and an end, but how people journey through it is an individual experience. It is a chaotic process with people swinging between realisation of the loss when the loss is felt strongly and times when it is difficult to believe the loss has occurred. It is frightening and unsettling. In time, however, the swing becomes less and people spend more and more time in recovery:

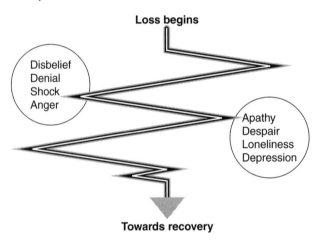

What feelings can occur?

When a life-threatening illness is diagnosed the patient, partner or relatives may go through many different feelings. They may go through these feelings intensely a second time when the patient dies.

Disbelief: some may feel shock at what the news is and any one of the family may react with numbness or denial at the reality.

Anger: others may react with anger or frustration that someone close is going to be taken from them, especially at the meaninglessness of the situation or its unfairness.

Anxiety about this new situation can result in fear with feelings of vulnerability and loss of security.

Guilt: any of the family may feel guilt, for example children can feel that it's somehow their fault, that if only they'd been good.

Sadness is to be expected, especially sadness at loss of the future with a yearning that things were different.

Pining for normality can occur with a mixture of many of the feelings already described.

Despair can intervene and may even lead to depression.

Excess activity can occur by 'keeping busy', and irritability and exhaustion can develop.

Grief: the loss of their future with their family and not being able to see their children grow up.

How can I use this information?

1 We can help partners and family in their bereavement in the weeks and months *before* the death. The patient becomes an important part of this bereavement care.
2 We can expect many different feelings as part of grief, although an individual tends to have a typical pattern of reaction.
3 At times grieving people will find it difficult to concentrate and make decisions and we need to take this into account when giving information or obtaining consent.
4 Grief gradually becomes less chaotic, slowly leading to recovery.

Key points

- Loss is a common experience that depends on our life experiences – we all react differently.
- Grief is a chaotic process where individuals swing between recovery and the intense feeling of loss.
- A wide range of responses to loss is possible and is similar in patients and relatives.
- The losses that end in bereavement start at diagnosis.

How can I support the patient, partner and relative?

What should I know?

Adjustments

As the end of life approaches the patient, partner, family and carers all have to make adjustments. Some small adjustments have been made over weeks or months, but as death approaches the reality of the situation sometimes makes adjustments more difficult. And those who have been putting these adjustments off may have to catch up rapidly.

Adjusting to loss

This is never easy. The loss that the patient, partner and family are now experiencing so strongly actually began at the time of diagnosis. People cope with loss by shuttling between denial and realism – this is normal. Most people do both – one minute someone may be arranging their funeral, while the next they are talking about next year's holiday! It is like travelling on a road with potholes and distant views – looking only at the potholes avoids tripping but lacks interest, whilst looking only at the views hopefully means missing the potholes.

Denial

This can seem abnormal at the end of life, but careful listening reveals that most people are being realistic (e.g. 'I do hope he can get well enough for that holiday, but he does look an awful lot worse.'). People need to adjust at their own pace and forcing the pace is unhelpful. So if the patient, partner and family are managing day-to-day activities, then they are coping and need our offer of support, not our interference! Denial is often a necessary and effective coping mechanism.

How can I use this information?

In the last days of life there are a number of aims uppermost in the minds of professional carers. These include the following:

1 Set realistic goals and anticipate changes.
2 Provide individualised care. Keep the patient, partner and family fully informed. This includes keeping them informed of changes and helping them to understand these.
3 Control symptoms, stop unnecessary drugs and continue necessary drugs by an appropriate route.
4 Ensure the environment is quiet and comfortable.
5 Give (and accept) advice and support.

If you feel at a loss, speak to your colleagues. Nobody has a library of the right things to say. Don't punish yourself for not making things 'better'. Being there, listening and giving explanations when asked will be the most help. Partners and relatives often say later that this simple help is what they found most comforting and helpful. If difficulties remain, your local palliative care team will be able to advise and help.

Drinking and feeding

The issue of patients' food and fluid intake causes professionals much concern.

* Feeding may give continuing pleasure and optimism to a patient and partner. Drinking keeps the mouth moist and helps to keep it clean. It also reduces thirst and may reduce the incidence of drowsiness, confusion and pressure sores.
* Some patients are too ill and/or exhausted to manage food. Feeding will bring no advantages when the deterioration is rapid (day by day or faster). Drinking

may be difficult or impossible. There are a number of other routes (intravenous, subcutaneous, nasogastric, gastrostomy), but all have their own problems of discomfort, cosmetic appearance and the need for monitoring.
- At the end of life, drinking and feeding have nothing to do with 'resuscitation', but everything to do with comfort. Do what the patient, partner and relatives together feel is best for them!

Medication

You will notice a number of drug changes being made towards the end of the patient's life. This is a time of continual review. The doctor and the key nurse will be seeing the patient at regular intervals during the day. In making changes the doctor thinks about the following.

Drugs that can be stopped: laxatives can be stopped if the patient has had a comfortable stool before the deterioration. Most people can mange for up to 2 weeks without a laxative.

Drugs that must be continued: drugs like morphine need to be continued, but by a different route. The subcutaneous route is the most common, but for convenience diamorphine is used since it is very soluble and can be used in low volumes.

Drugs that require regular review: steroids are usually stopped in a rapidly deteriorating patient, regardless of the length of previous treatment. In patients deteriorating more slowly, steroids are usually reduced slowly.

With sleeping tablets, unless these were started recently, an equivalent will need to be continued to avoid agitation due to withdrawal.

Cigarettes are rarely continued by very ill patients. Beware, however, of agitation due to nicotine withdrawal. This is treated with a nicotine patch.

Key points

- It is normal for patient, partners and family to swing between denial and realism – denial is often an effective coping mechanism.
- Don't punish yourself for not making things 'better'. Being there, listening and giving explanations when asked will be the most help.
- Decide about drinking and feeding according to what the patient, partner and family need and feel is right for them.
- Some drugs need to stop, others can continue.

How do I help with a dying patient's distress?

What should I know?

The following figure details problems which were reported in 200 patients during the last 48 hours of life.

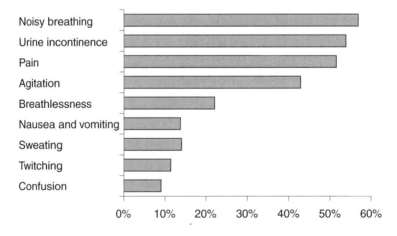

How can I use this information?

Noisy or rattley breathing does not necessarily cause distress for the patient but it is disturbing for relatives. It may be sufficient to change the position of the patient to reduce noise. Otherwise a drug called hyoscine butylbromide (Buscopan) can greatly help 50% of cases of rattley breathing. Gentle suction is occasionally needed.

Urinary incontinence (unable to control urine): urinary output often falls as the patient becomes more ill but the patient may still be incontinent. Various types of pads can help. For some patients a catheter might be introduced or sheaths for male patients. It is essential to maintain a dry, clean and healthy skin, and to help the patient with the distress they will feel at being incontinent.

Pain: the cause needs to be found. Consider an uncomfortable position causing muscular ache and pressure, or causes of pain such as urinary retention or constipation. It is necessary to ensure the patient's comfort and that the appropriate people are informed about pain and the effects of any medication.

Restlessness/agitation/confusion: once again the cause must be found and treated if possible. There may be emotional distress due to fear or low mood which needs to be addressed. Patients differ here, some may quieten in the presence of someone at the bedside whilst others might become more agitated or confused in the presence of people. Sedation is not routinely administered to dying patients, but it may be needed if they are very distressed. The patient's family will need reassurance and may also appreciate you staying with them until their anxieties settle.

There are a number of fairly simple things to try when a patient is agitated and confused. You can:

- switch on some indirect light
- gently and quietly explain what is happening to the patient (many confused patients can be helped to understand what is happening)
- make sure the environment is quiet
- keep visiting strangers to a minimum
- explain what is happening to partner, family and staff.

Confusion and agitation are likely to arise as a result of:

- drugs being started or stopped
- chest or urinary infections
- full bladder or rectum
- chemical changes in the blood.

Treatment can start if the patient and carer agree. The confused patient still has the right to refuse treatment (unless they are harming themselves or others). If the agitation is distressing to the patient, then it needs to be settled. Drugs are used depending on whether it is mainly fear that is the problem or abnormal experiences such as being suspicious of everyone.

Breathlessness: the cause needs to be found and treated. You might try some simple measures. Sit the patient upright, use a fan or open a window to get a cool airflow across the face. Relaxation and explanation will also help. The doctor might prescribe oxygen and perhaps drugs that will reduce fear. Family members feel less helpless if they are involved but they will also need some support.

Nausea/vomiting: the patient may already be receiving drugs to combat nausea and vomiting. The most appropriate route should be chosen to continue these. Simple measures are helpful such as mopping the forehead with a cool sponge or cloth, and having a bowl on hand in case of vomiting.

Sweating: keep the patient cool. Regular changes of bed linen and the use of cotton nightwear will help. This is a key area where you can involve relatives in sponging the patient. Drugs might be needed to help reduce night-time sweating.

Jerking/twitching/plucking is sometimes due to an excess of morphine in the system. It can also be caused by kidney failure or brain problems. If the patient is unsettled then gentle sedation may be needed. Relatives need explanation and reassurance here.

Key points

- A number of problems can cause distress in the last 48 hours.
- Most problems can be treated.
- All have simple treatments, which should be used first.

What do I do when a patient dies?

What should I know?

What happens to the patient?

For most patients with advanced illness there is a gentle 'winding down' of the body's systems. Even in cardiac and respiratory failure, sudden, dramatic deaths are uncommon. As they approach the end, their circulation slows so that their fingers, nose and toes feel cool and are a little bluish or mottled. Their breathing pattern may change and become slower or irregular. At the end it is more a gentle absence of life, than a sudden presence of death. Peaceful silence is the most obvious feature.

What happens to the partner and relative?

Those close to the patient respond differently. Some find it easy to cry, others feel as though they have dried up. Some feel the urge to speak, often to express relief. Others feel it's an anticlimax because, in a sense, the person left hours or days before. Many are so numbed with grief that they feel helpless and useless, but often will not admit to this. They cannot remember names, addresses and telephone numbers.

What happens to you

Professionals are also affected by the death of patients. *'Awkward'* is how it feels. There is an overwhelming feeling to do something – check the pulse, move a pillow, make tea, say something – usually something like 'Well he's at peace now'.

How can I use this information?

There are no rules, but there are some principles.

- Take your cue from the family or partner; enable them to do it their way.
- Silence is awkward, but is right in the right place (there's nothing you can say that will make it better).
- If those present want to talk then talk, if they're silent then let them be silent.
- If you're present whilst the patient is dying, you or a colleague should keep a check on a pulse point. Rather than state 'He's dead now', use phrases like, 'The pulse is very weak.' and 'I can hardly feel a pulse now.' This will prepare those present for the end and give you time to make sure it is the end since the pulse often slows gradually, rather than stopping suddenly.
- Someone will need to check that the patient has died. Don't pronounce death until at least 5 minutes have elapsed from the last breath (some patients take an occasional breath for several minutes).
- After the death, ask those present if they want to stay, and if so, do they want to be alone.
- Now go and make that cup of tea!

Other practical steps

The family may need help with practical arrangements. If so, this tends to make you feel better since there are things you can do! There may be family and relatives to contact. Find out what the plans are for a funeral or cremation and it may be helpful for you to make the initial phone call to the funeral director and to explain how to register a death.

The death certificate

The death certificate shows the cause of death (e.g. cancer of the breast) and not the mode of death ('respiratory arrest' or 'coma'). The doctor who saw the patient within the last few days should complete the certificate, then explain and answer any questions raised by the family. There is no reason to seal the certificate in an envelope, it is better for the relative or partner to see the certificate and have the words on it explained. Sometimes the patient or partner has requested that the diagnosis be kept from other relatives (e.g. in AIDS). In such cases the immediate cause of death is given and the box on the back of the certificate is ticked. The registrar then contacts the certifying doctor later for the underlying cause.

Post-mortem

If a post-mortem is needed the doctor will obtain consent and explain the arrangements. Post-mortems are required by law in death due to industrial disease (e.g. asbestosis), injury, neglect, suspicious circumstances, or within the normal recovery time of an operation. Post-mortems are also a valuable way of obtaining information. A relative's permission is essential and usually it is not difficult to ask if this is done sensitively (e.g. 'It would help us to examine . . . to find out why he had so much pain'), and it is made clear that the relative or partner can refuse. It is unusual for a funeral to be delayed by a post-mortem.

Belongings

If the patient has died in hospital or other institution you will need to ensure that the patient's belongings are handed over. This is always a difficult task because it marks the finality of the relationships with the patient, the family and staff members. Finally, enquire about arrangements for getting home. Although they may have made the journey by car the driver might not feel competent to drive home. Offer to arrange a taxi.

> **Key points**
> - For the patient at the end it is more a gentle absence of life, than a sudden presence of death.
> - Partners and families react in different ways – the key is to let them do it their way.
> - For the professional there is a feeling that there is much to be done, but just being there is the most important factor.
> - The partner and family need to be helped with arrangements, including the certificate and post-mortem.

Death of a patient's friend or relative

What should I know?

This can happen during any illness and is an added burden on the patient.

Death of a fellow patient

Many patients develop friendships with fellow patients through their shared experiences. This may be a recent friendship, such as with someone in the same bay in hospital or hospice, or may be over months through attending the same day hospice, or over years through living in the same community home. Regardless of the length of the friendship, the death of one patient can be a great loss for fellow patients.

The consequences of not sharing loss

Every person will experience loss and bereavement at some point in their lives, but many people shy away from discussions involving death and dying, and as a consequence these issues have become stigmatised by society.

Examples of this tendency to 'hide' death are:

- 'hiding' the body by shutting the door, closing the curtains or putting the body in a box designed to look like a trolley
- talking in whispers

- not telling children
- a determination to continue as normal
- not telling fellow patients
- moving the body as soon as possible.

This reluctance to share the loss results in fellow patients and staff suppressing their grief and having feelings of uncertainty, tension and fear. These problems occur because fellow patients and staff fail to view the death holistically from physical, psychological, social and spiritual points of view.

How can I use this information?

- **Honesty**: honesty is the place to start. Every person is an individual in their own right and their specific needs will vary, but more harm will come from hiding fellow patients from the truth.
- **Others suffer too**: fellow patients are as likely to suffer from the loss as anyone else. Taking time to sit and talk with a fellow patient can be very beneficial and this includes people with alternative communication.
- **Don't 'jolly'**: it should be remembered that it is quite normal to feel sad and hurt during a time of loss, it is unhelpful and potentially damaging to try to 'jolly' the person along.
- **Reflecting back**: for many people life-story work is a useful way to communicate significant life events, and can be seen as a vital element in helping the person bring back memories both good and bad that would otherwise be forgotten. The concept of life-story books is also acknowledged in bereavement counselling with literature explored.
- **Look for changes in behaviour, which might indicate difficulty in expressing an emotion**: don't assume that behaviour changes are a result of grief (they may be related to something else). Remember that for some people, a grief reaction may take time to manifest itself.
- **If memory is poor**: reinforce the loss to assess the understanding and feelings about the death. Repeat ideas often to encourage learning.
- **Adjustment to the change**: ensure help and support are given while the person is adjusting to living in an environment where their friend is missing.
- **Telling families**: families may not know how to break the news of death to their relatives, especially if they are very young or have learning disabilities; they may try to protect the person from the effects of grief, whilst unintentionally making matters worse. Often in cases where a parent has died, a child or person with a learning disability may have lost the person who understands

them most. Informing the person allows the carer to prepare them for their possible loss. Carers can test informally a person's understanding of the concept of death, and what it means to that person, by using issues raised on television as a starting point. Although a person with learning disabilities uses the words 'death'/'dead', this does not imply that they understand the concept. Keep ideas simple and concrete.

How do people with learning disabilities experience bereavement?

Historically it is believed that people with learning disabilities were not capable of understanding or expressing grief. Whether through ignorance or a misguided attempt to protect the person the death of a relative is often glossed over. Individuals are prevented from attending the chapel of rest or funeral following the loss of a loved one. Sometimes relatives and carers make a conscious effort to hide their true emotions from the person with a learning disability.

People with learning disabilities can suffer any of the normal reactions to bereavement. They may also have additional special difficulties due to poor intellect and complex needs, which deny them the many social, verbal, auditory and visual opportunities of realising that the death has occurred.

It is important to remember that people with learning disabilities have the same right to take part in family rituals as anyone else. These should include:

- receiving/sending cards
- sending flowers
- helping to choose hymns or poems.

Key points

- Death of a relative, friend or fellow patient adds an extra burden for patients.
- The consequences of hiding the loss are usually worse than being honest and supportive.
- People with learning disabilities react to loss in the same way as everyone else.

Supporting staff after a patient has died

What should I know?

About staff needs

Staff may be so involved in responding to the grief reactions of the remaining patients that their own feelings go unrecognised. The sheer workload in some teams prevents staff exploring what they feel about the death of a patient.

Permission to cry

Staff need 'permission to cry'. Some health teams understand this and allow staff to show their feelings, but other teams cannot cope with such emotion, viewing it as 'unprofessional', 'letting the team down' or even seeing it as a weakness. This may lead to feelings being hidden and possible problems not being addressed. Staff most commonly take their unresolved feelings home. Although they may share the reasons with their partners or family, it is more common for them to 'dump the feelings' on the unsuspecting partner or family without being able to explain the reason why. It will be harder if the staff member has recently had their own bereavement.

Reassurance

Care staff usually perceive themselves as being able to make things better so may feel they have failed in this situation. Guilt may be the result. This in-built desire to 'fix things' can prevent staff from realising that, in reality, they made a difference by being with the patient and family, and that this was therapeutic and helpful.

Organisational issues

Organisations should respect the needs of the patient/staff – remembering to leave an appropriate length of time before re-allocating the bed. In a busy health service, stretched at times beyond its ability to cope, this is not always possible, but a period of bereavement, however brief, should be the aim when possible.

Time to reflect on the situation

Now the roller-coaster has stopped; the staff need time to reflect on:

- the progression of the patient's disease
- the nature of the death (was it peaceful and expected, or was it unexpected or distressing?)
- how the death has impacted on both patients and staff.

Closure

This typically North American term describes the completion of a grieving process. Closure is difficult in many health settings and it is not possible to achieve it with every death. Attending the funeral or service of just one patient can act to 'close the chapter' on other deaths. Talking to bereaved relatives may also help.

Complications of staff bereavement

Staff denial

This works if the feelings are being channelled elsewhere, but may cause that member of staff to remain distant from the next dying patient for fear of exposing unresolved feelings.

Team denial

This can result in a team which is uncomfortable with dying patients, preferring instead to keep treatments going that are clearly no longer of benefit. Their discomfort will make it very difficult, if not impossible, to share the patient's fears or distress. Consequently they may miss problems that could be treated, such as depression, or may ask for the patient to be moved elsewhere, believing that this is the kindest thing to do.

Stress and burnout

Some stress is necessary for us to do our jobs well (it is possible to be *too* relaxed!). If this stress builds up because of blocked feelings then the staff member may eventually suffer from an anxiety state or clinical depression, along with physical symptoms of exhaustion, difficulty in making decisions, and feeling unable to come to work. They feel guilty that they haven't been 'stronger'. This is known as 'burnout' and usually catches people unawares since the sufferer is often the last to acknowledge that they are suffering from stress.

How can I use this information?

If there are team difficulties with emotions or death, don't try to sort this out yourself. This needs organisational change and education, neither of which can occur overnight or without the help of others.

In the meantime:

- find someone you can talk to about coping with patients' deaths – an understanding colleague at work is often better than taking the issue home and dumping it on your partner
- even if you can't cry with your team, find somewhere quiet and have a good cry, with a colleague if you can
- look back on the things you did that made a difference, keeping the patient comfortable, looking after the relatives. It's often the small things that make a difference
- try to go to one funeral of a patient – it often helps to 'close the chapters' of many other deaths. Don't be ashamed of using a funeral in this way – funerals are about the dead, but they are for the living.

Key points

- Staff can find it difficult to show their grief because of workload or team discomfort with emotions.
- Not addressing this grief results in staff keeping an emotional distance from dying patients, team difficulty in accepting the closeness of death and burnout for some individuals.
- You can take some simple measures to help yourself.

Complicated grief

What should I know?

We react to grief and loss in very different ways. People oscillate between experiencing loss and working towards restoration. In the early stages these oscillations are rapid and intense, gradually reducing over time and moving more towards restoration. The extent of these oscillations will depend on a whole host of past experiences, personality and current issues. Not surprisingly, therefore, it is not possible to talk about 'normal' or 'abnormal' grief. The one clear feature, however, is that most people find they begin to cope and function more effectively as time passes: 'It feels like you're stuck on an empty train that's stopped at an empty station. But trains move . . . .'.[1]

There are some people, however, who find it difficult or impossible to cope and function. They repeatedly oscillate back into experiencing loss. Their grief often becomes complicated by turning to alcohol or drugs, by developing psychological problems such as depression, anger, anxiety states or phobias, or by damaging existing relationships or developing unhelpful new ones. Any of these problems can affect the physical health of these individuals who may develop physical illness.

What helps or hinders the resolution of bereavement?

Factors which help resolution include close relationships, the perception of a good network of support, strong spiritual beliefs of any sort, a good relationship

---

1 Adapted from Lewis CS (1966) *A Grief Observed*. Faber and Faber, London.

with the person who died, a feeling of 'closure' about the life and death of the person (i.e. no 'unfinished business'), a peaceful and expected death, being present at the death and the healthy status of the bereaved.

Factors which can hinder resolution include poor relationships, little or no social support, a difficult or poor relationship with the person who died, 'unfinished business', difficulty in shedding tears, a sudden or unexpected death, a distressing death, being unable to fulfil a wish to be present at the death or funeral, illness in the bereaved, bad experiences of previous deaths, the presence of other sources of stress (e.g. recent divorce or death), lack of planning in financial or business affairs and absent or inadequate care arrangements for children.

All of these factors indicate a risk that bereavement may resolve slowly. Other risk factors include persisting anger or guilt, extreme or obsessive crying after the first few months, previous psychiatric history or suicidal tendencies and drug or alcohol dependence.

High risk factors: in reality, any factor could indicate a high risk in certain circumstances. For example, being absent at the time of the death is less of a risk if the bereaved person felt they had already said all that needed to be said. On the other hand, missing the opportunity to say goodbye or express their love could seriously hinder the resolution of their bereavement.

How can I use this information?

If it is obvious from discussion with relatives, and after acknowledging their feelings, that they may require further support/help to work through the bereavement process, use the following networks:

Clergy: support for the family could be gained both in the short and long term.

School staff: opportunities to discuss feelings and concerns with staff who have cared for any children.

Medical staff: support for the family and to discuss unresolved issues. The general practitioner is often the first line of help and should automatically be meeting the bereaved within a few weeks, and again after a few months.

Specialist help: persistent or complicated grief will need more specialist help from a bereavement service, counsellor or psychiatrist. The aims of counselling the bereaved correspond to the four tasks of grieving.

1 To increase the reality of loss.
2 To help the survivor come to terms with both his/her expressed and latent feelings.
3 To help with making the readjustments necessitated by the loss.
4 To encourage the survivor to make a healthy emotional withdrawal from the deceased and to feel comfortable reinvesting that emotion in another relationship.

The availability of these services depends on local resources.

Key points

- For some people grief takes longer to resolve and they are more severely affected.
- Many factors can hinder the resolution of grief, including unfinished business, an unexpected death or previous experiences.
- Support can be available locally, but the availability of specialist help depends on local resources.

Section 8
Spirituality and equality

- Fostering hope
- What is spirituality?
- How can I help someone with a different faith to mine?
- How can I avoid discrimination?

Fostering hope

What should I know?

Hope of realistically achieving something good in the future is at the heart of coping with advanced illness and enabling a good quality of life. Unlike denial or optimism, hope needs people to be realistic, since one can only successfully hope for something that is possible, not something that can never be achieved. It is about being open to possibilities.

What it is not

- It is not about being unrealistic.
- It is not the same as denial.
- It is different to optimism which needs denial and avoids reality.
- It is not about finding the meaning of life.

What it is

- A realistic desire for good in the face of uncertainty.
- It helps a person cope with tragedy and loss.

What hope needs

- A person to confront uncertainties, but at their own pace.
- Professionals willing to offer information at the person's pace, not the pace of professionals.

- Support the person can trust and feeling safe to express their distress.
- A willingness to consider possibilities.
- Professionals who are willing to allow and help a person to adapt their hope as their illness progresses.
- The ability of the person to imagine their hope by seeing it as a realistic possibility, not just fantasising or wishing that something may happen.

How does hope show itself?

Hope shows itself in different ways at different stages of illness:

- early in the disease – hope of cure
- as illness progresses – hope of control, hope of comfort
- at the end of life – hope of peace.

Hope shows itself in different ways in different people:

- some people are practical in their hope, e.g. hoping to avoid pain, tie up loose ends, go home to die
- others are more generalised in their hope, e.g. the hope to be at peace, to take 'each day as it comes', a hope of 'letting go' at the end.

How can I use this information?

- As an illness progresses people need to be allowed to change their hope, e.g. from cure to comfort.
  Action: allowing them to talk freely about their fears and hopes will help.
- Keep a look out for patients whose pace of change has been abrupt, e.g. being told their illness cannot be cured or treated.
  Action: these people will need extra time to mull over this new information, with a trusting ear to listen.
- A person may make it clear they do not want more information at present, e.g. 'I don't want to hear any more bad news'. This shows the person is in 'reality overload' and cannot take any more information right now.
  Action: make sure the team knows of the person's wishes.
- Hope is soon damaged by persistent physical symptoms, e.g. pain, nausea, vomiting.
  Action: make sure the team knows about the problem.

- Hope is very difficult to keep going in the presence of persistent psychological symptoms, e.g. anxiety, anger or a clinical depression.
  Action: let the team know if a person seems anxious, angry, frightened or withdrawn.
- Hope is difficult to start up if a person's life has been one of neglect, rejection or abuse.
  Action: these people will need time to talk to mull over future possibilities. They may need specialist help.

---

1 Allow people to talk.
2 Give people time to adjust.
3 Let the team know if the person makes it clear they want no more information.
4 Let the team know if the person is distressed.

Key points

- Hope is a realistic desire for something good in the face of uncertainty.
- Hope is not about denial or optimism.
- Hope changes as the illness progresses.
- A trusted listening ear is the most helpful support.

What is spirituality?

What should I know?

Many have tried to define spirituality and found it hard to describe it or list its features. Its simplicity contrasts with the profound effects it has on people.

Case study
A seriously disturbed 19-year-old man had been kept in various psychiatric units and given drugs for unpredictable and sometimes violent behaviour. He was very small and thin, allowing him to escape repeatedly through tiny gaps in windows and doors. Repeated episodes of abuse and abandonment during childhood had led to a life of alcohol and drug abuse before he was admitted into care.

New medication had allowed him to occasionally go on outings under close supervision. One visit was to a donkey sanctuary and half way through the visit he suddenly ran off. Fearing another escape his nurses chased after him. They found him in an enclosure with his arms around the neck of a donkey. Tears were running down the man's face. He was calm and settled for many weeks afterwards, and further visits continued to help control his outbursts.

What it is

Spirituality is about all those things that shape us and that 'make us tick'. It includes our values and our understanding of the meaning of life and our place in the world. It's about those things that touch us in a way that is not necessarily physical, for example when we see a beautiful sunset or hear a piece of music. It includes a sense of awe and wonder.

What it is not

It is wider than faith, organised religion, new age beliefs or alternative treatments although people do give expression to their spirituality in these ways and find them very helpful.

How do people express their spirituality?

- Through the way some express dignity in the face of so much loss in their lives.
- Through comfort and trust in relationships between carer and patient.
- The ability to live each day to the full and still experience joy in their lives in the face of suffering.
- The unspoken connection of understanding between two people.
- The use and enjoyment of art, music, or books.
- The unspoken connection of understanding between two people.
- The determination to make the best of the time left.
- The successful fostering of hope in spite of advancing illness.
- The marked peace and acceptance some people have as they approach the last hours of their lives.
- The strength of some patients to stay alive for an important family event.
- The ability to peacefully let go of life.

How can I use this information?

- Past experiences of spirituality can help in recognising when it is present, or when it is absent.
  Action: think back to experiences you may have had like the ones above, or ask a colleague about their experiences.
- Use all the ways of fostering hope you can.
  Action: see *Fostering hope*, pp. 161–3.
- Relaxation can help some people to feel at peace.
  Action: find out what helps a person to relax, e.g. quiet, music, a good book, getting away from it all.
- Touch is comforting and relaxing for some people.
  Action: find out if someone is available who is trained to give massage, reflexology or aromatherapy.
- Some find it easiest to express their spirituality through their religious beliefs.
  Action: find a religious leader who understands how to enable people to express spirituality.

- Goals in life are important milestones, achieving some of them can be deeply satisfying, giving a sense of completion.
  Action: find out if there any goals the person has.
- Spirituality can be encouraged in surprising ways, such as painting, playing music, working with clay, visiting an informal garden or a donkey sanctuary.
  Action: find out what the person enjoys, but also look for ways of helping them try out new experiences.

---

1 Reflect on your experiences of spirituality or those of others.
2 Foster hope.
3 Ask a religious leader for help if this is easiest for the person.
4 Explore surprising ways of encouraging spirituality.

Key points

- Spirituality can have profound effects on people.
- It is not the same as religion or belief.
- It can be seen in some people at different stages of their illness.
- Spirituality can be encouraged through fostering hope, relaxation, touch and exploring ways of achieving goals and trying new experiences.

How can I help someone with a different faith to mine?

What should I know?

Different faiths have different beliefs

Christianity

Christians believe in following the example of Jesus, who they see as the embodiment of a loving, just and personal God, and through whom lies the salvation of humanity. Death is linked to God's judgement. Consequently suffering can be seen as good, leading to healing and a deeper existence. Impending death is a time of looking towards the afterlife. Forgiveness and absolution are important rituals before death (the 'last rites').

Islam

Muslims believe that God (Allah) revealed the beliefs of Islam to Muhammed, an ordinary man who taught that all people were called to Allah's service and should live a good life. Muslims do not drink alcohol, do not eat pork or pig products, eat only specially prepared meat ('halal' meat), and only eat food that has been separately cooked and served. Death is seen as inevitable and that to struggle against it is wrong.

Judaism

Judaism developed from the religion of the ancient Israelites as recorded in the Hebrew Bible (the Old Testament) and given by God to Moses. Orthodox Jews believe in an afterlife, but this is a less common belief in non-orthodox believers for whom the emphasis is on this life. Jews do not eat pork, shellfish or any fish without scales or fins, and strict followers do not mix meat and milk. All meat must be specially prepared ('kosher'). Preserving human life is fundamental, and acceptance of death is viewed as giving up which is not acceptable.

Sikhism

A Sikh is a disciple of Guru Nanak who lived in the sixteenth century and emphasised involvement with family, friends and community. Sikhs believe in reincarnation and that the next life can be influenced by actions in this life.

Hinduism

This is an ancient religion, perhaps 4000 years old, based on three supreme Gods, Brahma, Vishnu and Shiva. Hindus practice in different ways, but all believe in reincarnation, that this life will influence the next, and that body, mind and spirit are inseparable. Death itself holds little fear and is seen as achieving freedom.

Buddhism

There are different forms, some brought by Bohidharma from India to China in AD 520. It does not acknowledge a personal god as creator, but believes in rebirth where everything changes and repeated good lives result in 'nirvana', or perfection. The body is a temporary vessel in this process.

Chinese customs

Confucianism is a philosophy about solving the practical difficulties of life while Taoism is about developing inner peace. Buddhism and the worship of ancestors is common. Fatalism about death is common.

How can I use this information?

Christians

Ensuring regular access to Church services will help some. For others, guilt at having 'lapsed' can be helped by calling a sympathetic priest or lay visitor who understands Christian theology as well as terminal illness and grief. There are no special rituals for the body, although many are placed face up with the hands across the chest. Funerals are arranged according to the relatives' or partners' wishes and both burials and cremations are allowed.

Muslims

The patient may need help to wash five times a day before prayer and will need to know the direction of Mecca. They need access to appropriate food. The surrender to death can surprise Western professionals, but this can result in a peaceful acceptance of what is happening. The family and community need to be able to pray by the bed. The preferred position is to be placed with the face to Mecca. After death the body can be touched only by Muslims, or by staff wearing gloves. The limbs are straightened, head turned towards the right shoulder and the unwashed body wrapped in a plain sheet. The family will perform any additional rituals. Only burials are allowed and these must be as soon after the death as possible, so any delay due to post-mortem may cause distress.

Jews

They need access to appropriate food and to observe the Sabbath. The Sabbath (Friday sunset to Saturday sunrise) may be observed by lighting a candle and orthodox Jews may not use equipment, including lights. Psalms are read and the dying person is encouraged to pray. After death people stay with the body for eight minutes to confirm death. Staff should not attempt to lay out the body. The son or nearest relative closes the eyes and mouth, places the arms at the side of the body and binds the jaw. Traditionally, the body is placed on the floor with feet towards the door, covered with a sheet, with a candle beside it and is never left alone before burial. There is resistance to post-mortems as it is preferred to leave the body intact. Cremation is allowed by non-orthodox Jews.

Sikhs

They need to wear, or be close to, their 'kangha' (hair comb), the 'kara' (steel bangle) and the 'kirpan' (symbolic, short and blunt dagger which may be a brooch or pin). The 'kaccha' are special shorts which are kept partly on in the bath or shower before a new pair is put on. Respect for these Sikh symbols is very important. The emphasis on community can mean that a large number of people attend to the patient. After death, a Sikh is cremated as soon as possible.

Hindus

Modesty and cleanliness involving routines such as bathing daily in running water are important. No Hindu eats beef, and many are vegetarian. There is a strongly spiritual approach to death helped by priests (pandits or brahmins). Cremation is the accepted form of funeral.

Buddhists

They need as much time and space for meditation as possible and may refuse drugs in order to remain fully alert. They will need reassurance that sedation will be avoided. Some will inevitably feel anger, fear or grief and may feel guilty at their lack of calm. It helps to assure them that this is common, but calling in a Buddhist 'bhikku' or sister can help.

Chinese customs

There are few rituals before death, but after death rituals and the funeral are very important, and the patient may want to be reassured that everything is organised. The body is washed an uneven number of times with special water. Incense is burned, and the body covered in wadding and dressed with a special garment.

How can I avoid discrimination?

What should I know?

It is difficult to believe that discrimination exists in healthcare if you are an 'average' person, i.e. aged below 65, white, British, Christian, physically able, employed, mentally stable, heterosexual, with a local or standard accent and able to understand what is happening around you. In reality, there is good evidence that some people find it harder than others to get access to healthcare.

The elderly

Older people, especially those over 75 years, often have multiple problems. It can be easy to assume that some of their problems are an inevitable part of old age so that there is no point in referral to specialists and investigations. Even when a treatable diagnosis is made, there can be a tendency to assume that age itself is a reason not to treat so that treatment is not offered.

Ethnic minorities

People from a different culture may have different beliefs, practices and language to health carers. They may not be given the information to know what is available, or find it difficult to express their preferences and concerns. It is easy to misunderstand the importance of some practices, especially if they seem to go against Western beliefs about equality of the sexes or freedom of choice.

Disability and mental illness

Physical disability can make it difficult to access the GP or outpatients; learning disability makes it difficult for health carers to understand their needs; and mental illness can mask physical illness. Assumptions are made about their ability to undergo investigations so some are blocked from accessing screening tests. Health carers can feel embarrassed or frightened by such people so that they find it harder to make reasoned decisions about how to help them. Even if a treatable problem is found assumptions are made about their inability to cope with treatment, or professionals make judgements that assume they have a poor quality of life.

Low socio-economic status

Poverty is still a major problem for some people in the UK in some areas. The poor struggle to find healthy food, suitable homes or even simple shelter. This day-to-day struggle prevents them from considering health prevention such as screening or knowing what health support is available.

Different lifestyles

Health carers sometimes struggle with understanding people with different lifestyles to their own. Same sex partners may not be given the same consideration as other partners. Patients with an addictive or criminal lifestyle may be thought of as less deserving of care. Even people who prefer alternative and complimentary healthcare may be viewed as odd.

How can I use this information?

- **Get the facts right**: if you are ignorant about a person's condition, faith, culture or lifestyle, then make it the responsibility of you and your team to find out the facts. The facts are invariably less strange than your imagination!
- **Give people control**: illness removes control and good palliative care aims to restore as much of that as possible. Patients will want to observe rituals and religious festivals in their own way, as well as having access to their own food. Many families and communities need to pray with the patient. Making these people welcome and giving them a single room can be very helpful.

- **Don't impose**: serious, advanced or terminal illness is not the time to be sharing your beliefs or prejudices.
- **Don't guess the quality of life**: there is good evidence to show that healthcare professionals are inaccurate in their assessments of a patient's quality of life. Some organisations are now recommending that clinical judgements should not be made on this basis.
- **Ask yourself what you can do, not what you can't**: it is not about how your care is restricted by the patient's beliefs and practices, but how you can empower them to make the most of their life.

---

1   Get the facts right.
2   Give people control.
3   Don't impose.
4   Don't guess the quality of life.
5   Ask what you can do, not what you can't.

Key points

- Discrimination in healthcare is a problem for many groups or individuals with cultures, beliefs and lifestyles that are different to those of most health carers.
- Getting the facts right is an essential first step.
- You can help by giving people control, not imposing your own beliefs, not trying to guess the quality of life and by looking at what you can do, not what you can't.

Glossary

Glossary

Words in *italics* have a description in this glossary.

Active listening	The core of good *communication* where the carer works hard to ensure that the environment of listening is right and that the patient's thoughts and feelings are explored and clarified.
Acute confusion	A type of *confusion* that develops rapidly over hours or days. It is often due to infection, drugs or abnormal blood chemistry.
Addiction	A situation where a patient develops a reliance on a drug or chemical. Contrary to popular relief it is rare in patients taking *morphine* for pain relief.
Adenocarcinoma	This is a cancer that has developed from a surface *tissue* that has *glands* in it, e.g. breast adenocarcinoma.
Adjuvant analgesics	Drugs which relieve pain in an indirect way, e.g. antibiotics in pain due to infection.
Adjuvant treatment	Use of one treatment, e.g. *radiotherapy*, in addition (as an 'adjunct') to another treatment (e.g. surgery).
Agitation	A distressing sensation of fear, often with *panic* and *confusion*.
Analgesic staircase	Shows how *analgesics* can be *titrated*, starting with weaker analgesics and moving step-by-step to stronger analgesics. Also known as the analgesic ladder.
Analgesics	Drugs that are used to treat pain, e.g. paracetamol, morphine.

Anger A natural reaction to fear or being wronged. May be part of *anxiety* or *depression*.

Anorexia A diminished *appetite* caused by cancer or cancer treatment.

Antiemetic A drug used to treat *nausea* or *vomiting*.

Anxiety Feelings of being apprehensive, tense or on edge.

Anxiety state A situation when persistent *anxiety* has been present for 2 weeks or more and has four or more anxiety features present such as fear, irritability, poor concentration, restlessness and sweating.

Appetite The sensation of wanting to eat. It is often reduced in *cancer*, or following surgery or *chemotherapy*. Severe reduction is called *anorexia*.

Apthous ulcer A painful mouth ulcer.

Bad news News that is difficult for a person to take on board because it is likely to mean a major, difficult change in their life.

Benign tumour A collection of *cells* with uncontrolled growth, but which do not spread to nearby and distant *tissues*. Any effects are local.

Bereavement The term used to define the *loss* we feel following the death of a person or pet.

Biopsy A test where a small piece of suspicious *tissue* is taken for closer examination.

Blood and lymphatic tissues These are *tissues* whose *cells* make up the *lymph nodes,* spleen, *bone marrow* and blood.

Body image Part of our *self-image.* It is how we see ourselves physically, e.g. thin, fat, handsome, ugly.

Bone marrow The inside of bones which contains *tissues* that produce the cells that make up blood (*red cells, white cells* and *platelets*).

Breakthrough pain Episodes of *pain* that break through regular *analgesics.* If only occasional it needs a single dose of a quick acting analgesic. If frequent, the regular analgesic needs to be increased.

Breathlessness A sensation of not being able to get enough oxygen into the body.

Burnout The final pathway of persistent and severe *stress.* The person can no longer function at work or home, often suffering a clinical *depression,* usually with an *anxiety state.*

Cachexia	A special process which causes the body to lose fat and muscle. Although it also reduces appetite, the weight loss is not due to starvation but to changes in the way the body handles food and energy. It can be caused by cancer, chronic infection and severe heart disease.
Cancer	A collection of *cancer cells* which have uncontrolled growth and the ability to invade other *tissues*.
Cancer cell	A *cell* which differs from normal *cells* in two ways: – it duplicates itself without restriction, causing uncontrolled growth – it has the potential to invade nearby *tissues* as well as travel to and grow in distant *tissues*.
Candida	A yeast which normally lives in the body, but can overgrow to cause *pain* and *inflammation*, usually in the mouth or vagina.
Carcinoma	This is a cancer that has developed from a surface *tissue*, e.g. skin carcinoma.
Cell	The building block of all *tissues* that contains our *genes* and makes each *tissue* function correctly. Cells are normally under tight control so that they produce *tissues* that are the right size and function.
Central nervous system	The main control centres of our nervous system: the brain, spinal cord.
Cervix	The entrance to the uterus (womb) which can develop a *cancer*. It is curable if found early.
Chemotherapy	Usually means treatment of *cancer* with drugs that have the capability of killing *cancer cells*.
Chromosomes	These are complex *proteins* which contain a series of *proteins* called *genes*. The special protein that forms *genes* is called *DNA*. Nearly all cells have chromosomes and they lie in a bag called the nucleus in the centre of each *cell*. When a *cell* duplicates itself, the chromosomes are also duplicated. Humans have 23 pairs of chromosomes.
Chronic confusion	A type of *confusion* that develops slowly over months or years. Examples are senile dementia and the dementia associated with Down's syndrome.
Closure	This typically North American term describes the completion of *grief*. Closure is difficult in many health settings and it is not possible to achieve it with every death. Attending the funeral or service of just one patient can act to 'close the chapter' on other deaths. Talking to bereaved relatives may also help.

Cognitive therapy	A treatment that can treat anxiety and depression and which gives the patient skills that reduce the chance of the problem returning.
Communication	Our way of letting each other know who we are, what we know, and how we feel about ourselves, other people and the world around us.
Confusion	A frightening situation for patients where they have difficulty concentrating and understanding what is happening. There are two types, *chronic confusion* and *acute confusion.*
Constipation	Present when a patient passes a hard or uncomfortable stool and complains of persisting fullness.
Corticosteroids	Useful drugs that have many uses in *cancer* and *palliative care.* They are most commonly used to reduce swelling around a *cancer* (and so reduce local pressure effects) or to increase appetite.
CT scan	This uses *X-rays* taken in multiple views of the body to build up a picture using a computer. CT = computerised tomography. Gives more detail of soft *tissues* than *X-ray.*
Dementia	A condition causing a steady loss of brain *cells* over the years. It occurs in some older people, but can occur in younger people and in occurs in people with Down's syndrome.
Denial	A common and effective coping mechanism we all use when faced with an important *loss.*
Depression	A persistent low mood for more than 2 weeks, more than half the time, has four or more depressive-related symptoms and which is a change from their usual mood.
Diarrhoea	Present when stool is very soft or liquid. Occasionally can be caused by a bowel blockage or by *constipation.*
Differentiated cancer cells	Normal *cells* are designed for a specific place and purpose, e.g. a heart cell. Although differentiated *cancer* cells grow in an uncontrolled way, most still look and function like normal cells.
Difficult news	Information that is different to what the person expects. It may be *bad news*, but its impact depends on whether the person finds it difficult to accept.
Difficult questions	Questions such as, 'How long have I got left to live?' are difficult because of the suddenness of the question, the bad news that may be in the answer and the discomfort for the professional.

Distress	The outward sign of a person's physical or psychological discomfort.
DNA	This is a special *protein* which makes up our *genes*.
Drowsiness	A sensation of sleepiness and difficulty staying awake.
Encephalopathy	An infection of the brain, usually in childhood, which can cause brain damage. This can affect communication.
Endoscopy	A flexible tube containing optic fibres can be inserted into any body cavity and the view from the tip of the endoscope can be viewed outside. It is used to examine tubes and cavities in the body, and can be used to take *biopsies*.
Epithelial tissues	These are *tissues* whose *cells* are on the surface (e.g. skin) or form the linings of hollow organs such as the bowel.
Escalating anger	An important danger sign when facing an angry person.
Euphoria	When a person is extremely happy. It can occur as a side effect of some drugs such as steroids.
External beam therapy	Treatment using a machine (linear accelerator) to deliver *X-rays* in an accurate dose and *field* to a cancer.
Fatigue	A sensation of tiredness or having insufficient energy to carry out activities.
Field	Used in *radiotherapy* to describe the area that is exposed to radiation.
Fine needle aspiration	A test where a small needle is put into a suspicious lump and a few *cells* are removed. These cells are then examined to see if they are *cancer cells*.
Fractionation	Used in *radiotherapy* to divide treatment into two or more sessions to allow normal *tissue* to recover.
Frozen terror	A severe form of *panic* that prevents a person moving or speaking. May be part of an *anxiety state*.
Genes	Genes are a series of *proteins* which form a code. This code determines the characteristics of every part of us, from the colour of our eyes to whether we are more, or less, likely to develop *cancer*. Our genes sit in collections of many thousands of genes called *chromosomes*.
Glands	Many *tissues* in the body are able to secrete substances that are essential for the body and its function. Many glands in tubes and cavities produce mucin which protects, lubricates and cleans the linings. Other glands produce other substances, e.g. breasts produce milk.

Grief	This describes the feelings of *bereavement*. It involves physical symptoms and distortions of thought and emotions.
Heredity	This is the way the characteristics of our father and mother (such as eye colour) are handed down to us.
Hope	A realistic desire for good in the face of uncertainty which helps a person cope with tragedy and loss.
Hormone therapy	Some *cancers* are dependent on the presence of natural *hormones* to grow, e.g. breast cancer, prostate cancer. Hormone therapy uses drugs that suppress these natural *hormones* and so stop or reduce *cancer* growth.
Hormones	These are *proteins* which influence many of the ways in which the body grows and functions. Oestrogen is an example. The growth of some *cancers* is influenced by hormones, e.g. breast cancer can be affected by oestrogen.
Ileus	Paralysis of the bowel caused by drugs or infection. Needs to be considered as a cause of *constipation*.
Immune system	This system fights infection and destroys any invading or foreign *cells*.
Inflammation	A process where *tissues* become swollen, reddened and painful. It can be caused by injury, *radiotherapy*, infection and problems with the body's *immune system*.
Laxative	Drug taken by mouth which treats or prevents *constipation* by ensuring the stool is kept soft.
Learning disability	A condition which causes a person to gradually lose the ability to learn effectively. If severe, professionals can find it difficult to understand what a person is trying to communicate.
Leukaemia	A type of *cancer* which can develop from white cells in the *blood and lymph tissues*.
Loss	The feelings we have when we lose someone or something important.
Lymph channels	Part of the lymphatic system. They carry a fluid called *lymph*, draining it through *lymph nodes* and eventually returning the fluid back to the blood.
Lymph nodes	One type of *lymphatic tissue*. Lymph nodes act as junctions for *lymphatic channels*, as well as a place where special *cells* that fight infection live.
Lymphatic tissues	*Tissues* in the body with two functions: – help to fight infection (*bone marrow, white cells* in blood, spleen and *lymph* glands)

	– drain *lymph* from the tissues through lymphatics and *lymph* glands). The lymphatic tissues are part of the *immune system*.
Lymphoedema	Blockage or damage to *lymphatic tissues* causes an accumulation of fluid, e.g. if the *lymph nodes* of the armpit are damaged, a swollen arm may result.
Lymphoma	A type of *cancer* which can develop from *lymphatic tissues*, e.g. Hodgkin's lymphoma.
Malignant tumour	A collection of *cells* with uncontrolled growth and the ability to invade nearby *tissues* as well as travel to and grow in distant *tissues*. Its effects are often widespread.
Mania	An extreme form of *euphoria* where patients may act very abnormally despite feeling that everything is wonderful. Can be caused by some psychiatric conditions and can occur as a side effect of some drugs such as steroids.
Markers	Usually used to mean chemicals produced by a *cancer* which can be detected in the blood.
Mastectomy	Surgical removal of the breast to remove a *cancer*.
Metastases	Sites where *cancer cells* have grown, having travelled from the original *cancer* (often through the blood or *lymph channels*). Also known as *secondary cancer*.
Morphine	An strong *analgesic* for treating some pains in *cancer*. It is safe when used correctly.
Mourning	The public face of *grief*.
MRI	Magnetic resonance imaging. Uses high energy magnetic fields to build up a picture of the inside of a body. Gives more detail than a *CT scan*.
Myeloma	A type of *cancer* which can develop from the plasma cells in the *blood and lymph tissues*.
Nausea	A feeling of wanting to *vomit*. Vomiting does not always occur.
Nerve	The electrical 'wires' in the body which transmit signals to and from the brain.
Nerve receptor	Structure in *nerves* that responds to chemicals, pressure or damage to produce an electrical signal along the *nerve*, e.g. pain receptor.
Neuralgia	A type of pain caused by *nerve* damage which continues long after the damage has stopped, e.g. pain after shingles.
Neurological tissues	These are *tissues* whose *cells* make up the brain, eyes, spinal cord and nerves of the body.

NSAID	Non-steroidal anti-inflammatory drug, e.g. ibuprofen, diclofenac.
Nutrition	What we need to eat and drink to keep healthy.
Oestrogen	A *protein* which is a *hormone*. Some female *cancers* (e.g. breast cancer) are dependent for their growth on oestrogen.
Opioids	Chemicals that lock onto opioid *receptors*. Direct *analgesics* such are codeine and morphine are opioids.
Osteosarcoma	A type of *sarcoma* which develops from bone.
Pain	An unpleasant, complex, physical and emotional experience perceived by us as pain.
Palliative care	Aims to provide support and enable patients to deal with distressing symptoms and the concerns they have associated with an advanced and progressive disease which cannot be cured. Provided by specialist teams with accredited training in palliative care.
Panic	A feeling of terror that something dreadful is about to happen. May be part of an *anxiety state*.
Paranoia	When a person is suspicious of others or of objects with no apparent reason for that belief. Common in *acute confusion* and some psychiatric conditions.
Permission to cry	Some teams find it difficult to allow either patients or staff to do this describing it as 'labile emotions' or 'unprofessional'. The result is poor care of dying patients and increased staff *stress*.
Phobia	An overwhelming fear when faced with a particular object or situation. May be part of an *anxiety state*.
Platelets	Small structures in the blood that ensure the blood clots properly to prevent bleeding.
Primary cancer	The original site of the *cancer*.
Prostate	Gland in men at the base of the bladder which can develop a slow-growing *cancer* that tends to *metastasise* to bone.
Proteins	These are important chemicals in the living *cells*. They form the main part of many living structures, including our *genes*.
Radioactive sealed sources	Used in *radiotherapy*. Treatment involves placing *radioisotopes* in a sealed container which is then placed near or inside a *cancer*.
Radioisotopes	Short-acting radioactive chemicals attached to molecules which will attach to specific *tissues*. The radiation they give off can then be seen by detectors.
Radiotherapy	The use of radiation to kill actively growing *cancer cells*. It can be given by *external beam therapy*, *radioactive sealed sources* or by injected *radioisotopes*.

Receptors	Chemical structures that act as 'locks' for a chemical 'key', e.g. opioids are a chemical key which lock onto opioid receptors. Once the key and lock fit together, the receptor's function is activated, e.g. pain relief.
Recurrence	*Cancer cells* that were not killed by treatment which then grow and restart the *cancer*.
Red blood cells	Cells that carry oxygen from the lungs to the tissues.
Sarcoma	This is a type of *cancer* which can develop from internal *tissues*, e.g. *osteosarcoma*.
Screening	These are tests or investigations which search for the early signs of a disease so that it can be treated early. This is particularly important for *cancer* since many cancers can be cured if found early enough.
Secondary cancer	Sites where *cancer cells* have grown, having travelled from the original *cancer* (often through the blood or *lymph channels*). These sites are known as '*metastases*'.
Self-image	A person's own impression of their physical appearance, and what sort of person they feel they are, something which may or may not be accurate. An example is *body image*.
Side effects	Unwanted actions of medical or surgical treatments, e.g. a dry mouth from a drug to treat hay fever.
Spirituality	A profound change which can provide a peace and comfort at times of tragedy and loss. It is not about religion or faith.
Staff bereavement	Needs to be addressed and acknowledged if dying patients are to receive good care.
Stem cells	These are *cells* that have the ability to change into several different types of cells. They are found in the early embryo stages of development and in the *bone marrow.*
Steroids	Most commonly used in the form of *corticosteroids* in *cancer* and *palliative care*. Body building 'anabolic' steroids are not usually used.
Stress	Some stress is necessary and normal, but too much for too long results in *burnout*.
Supportive care	The universal form of *palliative care* that is the right of every patient and the duty of every professional.
Thrush	An infection caused by *Candida*, usually in the mouth or vagina.
Tissues	A collection of *cells* that has a specific function in the body, e.g. heart tissue, liver tissue.
Titration	The method of adjusting the strength and dose of a drug to suit an individual patient. Commonly used for *analgesics*.

Toxins	Chemicals that cause harm to the body.
Tumour	A collection of *cells* with uncontrolled growth: – a *benign tumour* does not spread to other *tissues* – a *malignant tumour* has the ability to invade nearby and distant *tissues*.
Ultrasound	High frequency sound waves are directed at the area to be examined through a layer of gel applied to the skin. The reflected sound waves are used to build up a picture of the internal structures. Detail is poor, but it is simple and can be arranged quickly.
Undifferentiated cancer cells	Normal *cells* are designed for a specific place and purpose, e.g. a heart cell. Undifferentiated *cancer* cells do not look and function like normal cells.
Vomiting	Bringing up the contents of the stomach. *Nausea* is usually present before vomiting.
White blood cells	Cells that are part of the *lymphatic system.* They are present in the blood and many *tissues*. One of their main jobs is to help fight infection.
WPC	Warn, Pause, Check. Three essential steps in breaking *difficult news*.
X-rays	Energy waves that can go through the body and leave a shadow of what is inside on photographic film placed behind the body.

Index